Portfolio Guidance for Veterinary Nurses

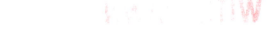

Senior commissioning editor: Mary Seager
Editorial assistant: Caroline Savage
Production controller: Anthony Read
Desk editor: Angela Davies
Cover designer: Alan Studholme

Portfolio Guidance for Veterinary Nurses

The College of Animal Welfare

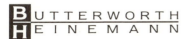

BUTTERWORTH
HEINEMANN

OXFORD   AUCKLAND   BOSTON   JOHANNESBURG   MELBOURNE   NEW DELHI

Butterworth-Heinemann
Linacre House, Jordan Hill, Oxford OX2 8DP
225 Wildwood Avenue, Woburn, MA 01801–2041
A division of Reed Educational and Professional Publishing Ltd

 A member of the Reed Elsevier plc group

First published 2000

Photograph by Mary Seager.
Cover photograph courtesy Aylmer & Cannon Veterinary Practice, Chipping
Norton, Oxfordshire, UK with grateful acknowledgement to Vanessa Bennett
and Kate Ormston.

British Library Cataloguing in Publication Data
Portfolio guidance for veterinary nurses
   1. Veterinary nursing – Great Britain – Examinations – Study guides
   I. College of Animal Welfare
   636'.089'073

ISBN 0 7506 4809 0

All information correct at time of printing

Composition by Genesis Typesetting, Rochester, Kent
Printed and bound in Great Britain by Biddles Ltd,
Guildford and King's Lynn

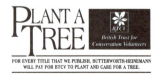

Acknowledgements

The College of Animal Welfare is most grateful for the help of the following colleagues in the preparation of this book: Barbara Cooper, Deborah Gould, Jessica Hargreaves, Andrea Jeffery, Hilary Orpet and Louise Tartaglia.

Contents

Introduction

In January 1999 the Royal College of Veterinary Surgeons (RCVS) Veterinary Nurse Training Scheme changed and became focused around Scottish/National Vocational Qualifications (S/NVQs). The aim of the change was to develop national standards for veterinary nursing, thereby improving the skills of the workforce and facilitating an improved standard of nursing care and practice.

Each student is required to develop a portfolio as evidence of the standards they achieve during their training as a veterinary nurse. This portfolio is used to provide evidence that they have achieved the occupational standard required for the S/NVQ in Veterinary Nursing, as well as acting as a suitable reference for future employers of veterinary nurses and as a record for continuing professional development as a qualified veterinary nurse.

The aim of this book is to support the documentation produced by the RCVS and thereby assist student veterinary nurses (SVNs) in the completion of the portfolio and help those involved in their training and assessment.

1 History of veterinary nurse training and assessment

Since 1961, when the first training and assessment programme for veterinary nurses was launched on a national basis, over 6400 students have qualified as veterinary nurses. Originally known as 'registered animal nursing auxiliaries' (RANA), the title was changed in 1984 to that of 'veterinary nurse' when a change in legislation removed the protection of the title 'nurse', originally only permitted to be used by members of the General Nursing Council.

Occupational standards for veterinary nursing have been developed and piloted by the Veterinary Lead Body since 1993, the aim being to develop standards that reflect the roles and responsibilities of the veterinary nurse, and outline those required for competent performance. Development of the standards was achieved through consultation with representatives of the veterinary and veterinary nursing professions.

Methods of assessment were then developed with the aim of maintaining the rigour of the existing professional examination whilst including practice-based assessment of performance and knowledge. This led to the development of the objective syllabus and practice portfolio.

2 The new veterinary nurse scheme

The new scheme is based upon practice training and assessment combined with an independent examination-based assessment (i.e. the RCVS VN examination). It normally takes 2 years to qualify as a veterinary nurse and this now leads to the S/NVQ at levels 2 and 3 when completed.

2.1 Enrolment

The following are the current requirements laid down by the RCVS for enrolment on the Veterinary Nurse Scheme:

- Be a minimum of 17 years of age.
- Hold a minimum of 5 GCSEs at grade C or above (or equivalent, e.g. the Pre-Veterinary Nursing Certificate). These must include English Language and either two science subjects or a science subject and Mathematics.
- Be employed at a practice that is an Approved Training and Assessment Centre (ATAC), or be a student on a Veterinary Nursing degree course.

2.2 Training

The student veterinary nurse (SVN) must be employed at an ATAC for a minimum of 94 weeks (full-time employment), including annual leave and sickness absence. Full-time employment should be considered as no less than 35 contracted hours per week (not to include on-call hours and overtime).

Part-time employment should equate to a minimum period of 165 weeks, including annual leave and sickness absence. Part-time employment should be considered as no less than 20 contracted hours per week (not to include on-call hours and overtime).

SVNs may choose to support their training in practice with educational courses, which may be full-time block release courses, part-time day release courses or distance learning programmes. The RCVS emphasize that, although it is not a mandatory requirement of veterinary nurse training, educational programmes that provide underpinning knowledge for the S/NVQ are recommended. They assist the student with the theory relating to practice, which in turn should improve the quality of nursing care and help the student achieve competence for the S/NVQ assessment.

2.3 Assessment

2.3.1 Practice-based assessment

Each student veterinary nurse is assessed on different activities within the ATAC. These activities are those detailed in the occupational standards and are recorded in the portfolio as evidence that the national standard has been met.

2.3.2 Independent assessment

This consists of:

- A written examination (consisting of two papers of multiple choice questions), which takes place during Part 1 training (towards the S/NVQ Level 2) and at the end of Part 2 training (towards S/NVQ Level 3).
- A practical examination of key practical skills which is taken at the end of Part 2 training (towards S/NVQ Level 3).
- External verification of the practice portfolio, which occurs in two stages, these being on completion of portfolio modules 1–5, i.e. NVQ Level 2 (Part 1), and on completion of modules 6–14, i.e. NVQ Level 3 (Part 2).

The RCVS administer all aspects of the independent assessment.

2.4 Qualification

The student achieves the S/NVQ Level 2 on successful completion of portfolio modules 1–5 and the Part 1 examination.

They complete S/NVQ Level 3 on successful completion of portfolio modules 6–14 and the Part 2 written and practical examinations.

Only following successful completion of S/NVQ Levels 2 and 3 does a student qualify as a veterinary nurse and become eligible to enter their name on the RCVS list of veterinary nurses.

3 Scottish/National Vocational Qualifications

3.1 History and structure of S/NVQs

In order to fully appreciate and work with the Veterinary Nursing S/NVQs it is necessary to become familiar with the structure and function of S/NVQs as a whole.

S/NVQs are qualifications based upon occupational standards developed by industry representatives. In the case of veterinary nursing, the standards were developed by the Veterinary Lead Body, which is composed of veterinary, veterinary nursing and allied industry representatives.

The Veterinary Lead Body conducted a detailed analysis of the sector and the job roles therein. From this analysis they were able to determine the main roles and responsibilities of the veterinary nurse and develop standards reflecting these roles. These standards show the outcome of competent performance, including the knowledge and understanding required to achieve the outcome.

The standards are composed of a number of different *units*, which represent key roles of the veterinary nurse. Each unit is further broken down into *elements* which are each composed of *performance criteria* (what the veterinary nurse should be able to do) and *knowledge and understanding* (what the veterinary nurse needs to

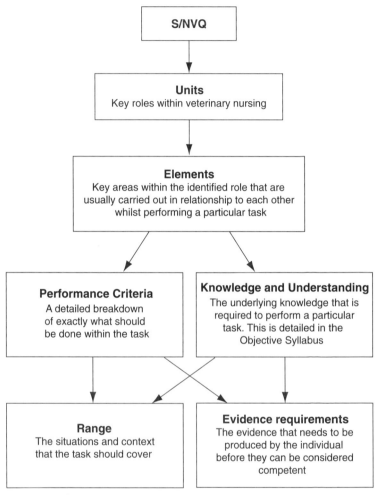

Figure 3.1 Structure of the Veterinary Nursing S/NVQs

know and understand relating to the element). This can best be represented by Figure 3.1.

S/NVQs can exist at Levels 1–5, although in the context of veterinary nursing at the time of writing, they are available at Levels 2 and 3. The level of the S/NVQ is defined by the responsibilities of the job role as detailed below:

Level 1 Work requires the person to perform a range of routine activities under supervision.

Level 2 The person is required to perform a range of routine and non-routine activities within their work, with limited supervision.

Level 3 The job role requires performance of a wide range of skilled and complex tasks and also includes responsibility for the supervision of others.

Level 4 Operating at managerial level, with the responsibility for controlling staff and resources.

Level 5 Operating at a senior professional level and being responsible for planning, policy development and the strategic management of the organization.

To qualify as a veterinary nurse, eligible for entry on the RCVS veterinary nurse list, students (or candidates – the terminology used for an individual working towards an S/NVQ) must complete Levels 2 and 3 of the Veterinary Nursing S/NVQ.

3.2 Accrediting and awarding bodies

Once occupational standards have been finalized by the Occupational Lead Body, e.g. the Veterinary Lead Body, they are submitted to the accrediting body for approval as S/NVQs. The accrediting bodies are:

- The Qualifications Curriculum Authority (QCA) for NVQs in England, Wales and Northern Ireland.
- The Scottish Qualifications Authority (SQA) for SVQs in Scotland.

These should not be confused with the awarding body, which, in the case of veterinary nursing, is the RCVS. As an awarding body the RCVS is responsible for the development and review of assessment systems, maintenance of quality assurance of the qualification, administration and certification procedures and marketing and promotional activities. They are also responsible for the approval of centres to offer the S/NVQs. These centres are known as Approved Assessment and Training Centres (ATACs) and are required by the RCVS to have access to a range of resources, a sample of which can be found in the *RCVS Training Centre Handbook* (details of where to obtain this are given in Appendix C).

4 Key roles and responsibilities in the delivery of S/NVQs

4.1 The people involved

Candidate: The candidate is the term given to the individual undertaking the S/NVQ. They have to be able to demonstrate that they are competent with regard to the occupational standards. In the context of veterinary nursing, the candidate is the student veterinary nurse who is working towards their S/NVQ Levels 2 and 3 in Veterinary Nursing.

Assessor: The assessor is the individual who assesses the candidate against the occupational standards to determine competency. In some situations there may be more than one assessor per candidate. The assessor should monitor the candidate's progress throughout the S/NVQ by planning assessment strategies and identifying assessment opportunities within the workplace. They should also help identify appropriate training for the candidate to assist them in achieving the occupational standards.

Internal verifier: The internal verifier (or IV) is the individual responsible for checking that the assessor or assessors are assessing consistently and fairly (between different candidates and assessors) against the occupational standards. They will usually be within the same practice as the assessor(s) although, where this is not possible, an IV from another practice may be enlisted solely to carry out internal verification duties (see also 4.3.2.)

External verifier: The external verifier (or EV) is employed by the awarding body, the RCVS. They are responsible for approval of centres (ATACs) and for verifying the assessment and verification decisions made by the assessors and internal verifiers from centres around the country, thereby ensuring that the standard is consistent between centres.

4.2 Assessment

In order to deliver the S/NVQs, all ATACs must have access to appropriately qualified and trained assessors, to assess the student veterinary nurse (SVN) against the occupational standards to determine competence.

The QCA/SQA and the RCVS determine require-ments for assessors. To be an assessor for the Veterinary Nursing S/NVQs the individual must:

- be a qualified veterinary nurse, whose name is maintained on the list held by the RCVS; or
- be a veterinary surgeon (MRCVS).

Each assessor should also hold, or be working towards, units D32 and/or D33 from the Training and Develop-ment S/NVQ of the Training and Development Lead Body (TDLB; now part of the Employment National Training Organisation).

These units are an important part of the S/NVQ assessment procedure. They provide evidence that the assessor is trained to assess candidates' performance (unit D32) and/or assess candidates using differing sources of evidence (unit D33) in a fair and consistent manner. They are a requirement of all assessors who assess S/NVQs, no matter what the occupational role.

4.2.1 Responsibilities of the assessor

The assessor is responsible for planning and conducting assessments with the SVN (or candidate) and maintaining accurate records of all such assessments. They should provide feedback to the SVN regarding their assessments and help to implement an appropriate corrective action plan should the standard not have been achieved on assessment. They should regularly review and monitor the progress of the SVN, discussing and agreeing any changes to the student's individual assessment plan that may be necessary. They should assist the SVN with the collection and presentation of evidence in the portfolio to support the assessment procedures.

4.3 Verification

There are two forms of verification, internal and external.

4.3.1 Internal verification

The internal verifier (or IV) usually comes from within the ATAC itself. In some circumstances the IV may be external to the ATAC and be employed by the ATAC to come in when necessary to carry out the internal verification procedures required by the RCVS.

The QCA/SQA and the RCVS determine requirements for IVs. To be an IV for the Veterinary Nursing S/NVQs the individual must:

- be a qualified veterinary nurse, listed in the RCVS Veterinary Nurse Register; or
- be a veterinary surgeon (MRCVS).

Each IV should also hold, or be working towards, unit D34 (and preferably units D32 and/or D33) from the Training and Development S/NVQ of the Training and Development Lead Body (TDLB; now part of the Employment National Training Organisation).

This unit (unit D34) is an important part of the S/NVQ verification procedure. It provides evidence that the IV is trained to internally verify the assessment process in a fair and consistent manner. It is a requirement of all IVs who verify S/NVQs, no matter what the occupational role.

4.3.2 Responsibilities of the internal verifier

The IV is responsible for the verification (checking) of the assessment practice of assessors. They should sample evidence from all assessors, ensuring that they cover all different forms of assessment used to verify the competence of candidates. During this process they should maintain accurate records of their internal verification. They are also responsible for liaising with assessors, identifying any training needs and co-ordinating the activity of the assessors within the ATAC through regular update meetings. They are also the first point of contact with the external verifier for the ATAC.

4.3.3 External verification

The external verifier (or EV) is employed by the RCVS to carry out external verification procedures across a number of ATACs on a national basis.

The QCA/SQA and the RCVS determine requirements for EVs. To be an EV for the Veterinary Nursing S/NVQs the individual must:

- be a qualified, listed, veterinary nurse; or
- be a veterinary surgeon (MRCVS).

Each EV should also hold, or be working towards, unit D35 from the Training and Development S/NVQ of the Training and Development Lead Body (TDLB; now part of the Employment National Training Organisation).

This unit is an important part of the S/NVQ verification procedure. It provides evidence that the EV is trained to externally verify the assessment process in a fair and consistent manner. It is a requirement of all EVs who verify S/NVQs, no matter what the occupational role.

External verification by the RCVS ensures that all veterinary nursing portfolios meet a minimum standard regarding the evidence contained. The EV examines case log sheets and other material to ensure that sufficient evidence has been supplied to support the assessor's decision that the SVN has met the national standard.

4.3.4 Responsibilities of the external verifier

The EV is responsible for monitoring the activities of ATACs on a national basis. They sample assessment practice and evidence to ensure that the standards are being met. This may involve direct observation of assessments and portfolios as well as discussions with SVNs, assessors and the IV. On completion of the appropriate modules of the veterinary nurse portfolio, the EV verifies the modules before the S/NVQ can be achieved. They are responsible for sampling the ATACs' internal verification methods as a means of quality control for the qualification.

EVs are responsible for supporting the ATAC during the initial implementation of the S/NVQs and subsequently advising as and when the need arises. They may choose to hold workshops for IVs and assessors to assist with this process and to provide networking opportunities for ATACs.

5 The veterinary nurse portfolio

The portfolio was introduced by the RCVS to assist both the SVN (candidate) and the assessor in the collection of evidence towards the Veterinary Nursing S/NVQs and should be used in conjunction with the occupational standards in the *Training Centre Handbook.*

It should be borne in mind that the nature of the portfolio and the diversity of veterinary practices will naturally produce different styles of portfolio. This is taken into consideration during the external verification process.

5.1 Portfolio structure and content

The portfolio is divided into a number of annexes with an introductory section including guidance notes and an index. It should be accompanied by a set of the occupational standards and the objective syllabus.

Throughout the portfolio there are some sheets that are laminated. It is intended that these are treated as master copies and photocopied before writing on them.

A portfolio coversheet should be completed with the relevant details, including name, enrolment number and date of enrolment. This forms the front page of the portfolio modules submitted to the RCVS for external verification.

Each page of the submitted portfolio should be numbered and recorded on a contents sheet. This provides an easy point of reference and is useful for cross-referencing.

A personal profile of the candidate should be completed and submitted as part of the portfolio. This should include details of the employment history and college-based training undertaken.

A signature authentication sheet should be completed by all those signatories in the portfolio including assessors, evidence gatherers (if appropriate) and the principal of the practice. It is advisable to complete this sheet as the SVN progresses through the portfolio. Should a member of the practice leave who has been involved with the portfolio without signing this sheet, it could take some time to track them down for an authentication signature.

Action plans should be completed initially and reviewed and updated regularly. This provides an opportunity for the assessor and SVN to plan evidence gathering and assessment. This is a working document and it should be reviewed regularly. Obviously there may be some situations where planned evidence gathering and assessments may be delayed – perhaps due to a particularly busy period within the surgery. This should be indicated on the plan and the action rescheduled for a later date.

The case log sheets for the different modules of the portfolio are designed so that they may be photocopied before use. The portfolio is available on the Internet from the RCVS for those students who wish to word process their evidence.

The Level 2 modules include:

- Basic Animal Management
- Communications
- Basic First Aid
- Human First Aid
- Dispensing Record

The Level 3 modules include:

- Laboratory Techniques
- Fluid Management
- Medical Nursing
- Radiography
- Surgical Nursing – General
- Surgical Nursing – Theatre Practice
- Anaesthesia
- Other Species – Exotics
- Health and Safety

In addition to the case logs, some modules require the completion of written reports or case studies.

6 General guidelines for the veterinary nurse portfolio

6.1 All sheets should be presented either wordprocessed, typewritten or neatly hand-written in blue or black ball-point pen (pencil is not a permanent record).

6.2 Any client details (name and address) should be removed to protect client confidentiality (therefore these should not be used for case number identification). Case number identification should be via the practice reference; however, where this is the client details then a suitable alternative should be used. A copy of the chosen method of log referencing relating to client details should be maintained (which should not be submitted with the portfolio). This will allow the candidate to relate back to original practice records if required, e.g. for completion of the Level 3 modules of the portfolio.

6.3 Evidence from the treatment of large animals (equines and farm animal species) should not be used within the portfolio, unless this is for neonatal care.

6.4 Where necessary, to avoid the duplication of information, appendices may be used and cross-referenced between case logs (but only where relevant).

E.g.   When considering the use of appendices in the Basic Animal Management (BAM) case logs:

Appendix BAM 1.1   Cleaning Protocol

could be used in the first BAM case log and referred to in subsequent logs where appropriate

Appendix BAM 1.2   Bedding Protocol

As above.

6.5 Each log sheet should have the name of the SVN, the SVN signature and the enrolment number and be signed and dated by the assessor when competency has been achieved.

6.6 Evidence can be recorded in sentence form or as bullet points, as long as major points are clarified. Consideration should be given to the space provided and clarity of presentation. Large quantities of 'waffle'/ irrelevant information is not considered appropriate. Where necessary, an additional sheet, firmly attached and neatly and clearly laid out with the appropriate heading and numbering, should be used. If additional sheets are attached, these should be recorded at the bottom of the case log sheet to prevent them being overlooked or misplaced.

6.7 Where a reference to a particular drug is made within the evidence of any unit (case log or written report), the generic name should be used. The only exception to this may be in the communication module, where for ease of client understanding it may be considered appropriate to use trade names only of wormers/flea treatments. If this is so, then the reason for this should be recorded in the case log.

6.8 'Student comments' should include the role that was played by the student in the case, e.g. sole charge for nursing care, and any other relevant information that the student may wish to contribute, such as general observations made by the student. 'Student comments' should be judged by the assessor. A meaningful short sentence should be encouraged.

6.9 The assessor's statement should indicate how the assessor came to the conclusion that the student was competent, i.e. a brief meaningful comment on the student's performance. This will need reference to the occupational standards in the handbook. The assessor may state that they questioned the candidate on an aspect of the log sheet and that these questions were answered correctly. This indicates evidence of knowledge and understanding.

7 Guidance notes for modules 1–5

7.1 Basic Animal Management (BAM) – Section 1

7.1.1   A separate diary is not necessary for this unit. The only evidence that is required is a completed log sheet.

7.1.2   Special care can be defined as any animal requiring observation between the parameters of normal and intensive care. In reality, with only a few exceptions (e.g. those healthy animals brought in by the general public as strays, awaiting re-homing or collection), the majority of animals within a veterinary surgery can be considered special care. The aim is for the student to include the most interesting cases that require 'specific' or 'special' nursing care. Recumbency, physiotherapy, basic wound management and hand feeding are possible examples. These may also be useful evidence for later modules in the portfolio.

7.1.3   Exotic species that are hospitalised may be considered as special care.

7.1.4   The student should demonstrate appropriate grooming of animals (cleaning, combing and brushing) during their stay within the case log sheets. Should a particular case not require grooming for a particular reason, then the student should state the reason(s) for this.

7.1.5   Timescale for treatment should include important features of the animal's stay, e.g. date admitted, date of any surgery, date discharged. There is no requirement to enter into detailed drug charts at this level.

7.2 Communication (COM) – Section 2

7.2.1   'Possible policies and approaches':
The choice of presentation style (e.g. size of leaflet, use of colour/pictures/diagrams, bullet points or sentences) relating where possible to ease of communication, should be included.

The production of a leaflet may be used to illustrate these points; however, if it is preferred, the student may include these by completing a detailed log sheet.

This section should also be used to outline the varying options that may be available, both within and between practices, relevant to the leaflet, e.g. use of different wormers/flea treatments, different ages for vaccination, different methods of control of oestrus, conducting ovario-hysterectomy before/after first season etc.

7.2.2   'Practice policy':
This section should be used to outline the practice policy within the ATAC.

7.2.3   See COM guidelines: 'the candidate should communicate verbally to owner . . .' witnessed by assessor.

7.2.4   Knowledge of the subjects in the communication section will be assessed in the independent assessment (examination).

7.2.5   'Post-operative care for routine operations':
This section relates to general information required for post-operative care and should include more commonly encountered post-operative situations, e.g. care of dressings.

7.2.6   'Dietary management of the normal animal':
This section relates to dietary management through the different life stages from puppy to old/geriatric.

7.2.7   The leaflet subject areas can apply to any species covered in the syllabus, unless specified in the guidelines.

7.3 Basic First Aid (BFA) – Section 3

7.3.1   The emphasis in this unit should be on BASIC First Aid.
Remember the three aims of first aid:

1. To preserve life.
2. To prevent suffering.
3. To prevent the situation deteriorating.

Therefore, simply by applying pressure (via a dry swab/gauze) to prevent further blood loss is basic first aid.

7.3.2   The first aid procedure should be described, which can be in brief using bullet points, for example when there is the need to describe the procedure for applying a dressing.

7.4 Human First Aid (HFA) – Section 4

7.4.1   Refer to the three aims of first aid in 7.3.1.

7.4.2   The most commonly encountered first aid incident is likely to be an animal bite to the SVN, VN or veterinary surgeon.

7.4.3   The assessor should decide how this should be assessed and may consider simulation of a first aid scenario.

7.4.4   Remember that for this unit the first aid incident does not necessarily have to be handled by the student. They are only required to be present and able to observe/assist.

7.5 Dispensing Record (DR) – Section 5

7.5.1   Some suggestions for your consideration that should be included – but only if they are applicable to the drug being dispensed and only if you carried it out:

- If the owner is instructed not to exceed the stated dose and/or not to use any other medication, then this could be included under Health and Safety (H&S).
- If the drug was dispensed in a childproof bottle, then this can be included under H&S.
- If the owner is instructed about storage of the drug, then this should be mentioned.
- If a penicillin-type drug is being dispensed, then the owner should be informed about penicillin sensitivity and instructed to wear

gloves if necessary – this can be included under H&S.

● Mention whether the owner is instructed to give the tablets with/without food, or whether they are told it does not matter.

● If tablets are required twice daily, then the owner should be instructed as to the timing of the doses, i.e. equally spaced. It should be recorded that you have informed the owner about this.

Common mistakes:

● Abbreviations, e.g. Prescription Only Medicine (POM), should be in full in the first instance. It is then satisfactory to use the abbreviation subsequently in one particular case log.

● Include both dispensing class, e.g. POM, and prescribing group, e.g. non-steroidal anti-inflammatory.

● In dose rate calculations always remember to put *mg per kg body weight.*

● Check that the duration of the course corresponds with the dates of treatment – if there is a reason why it does not, then explain why. This is likely to be an area to which the external verifier's attention may be drawn.

● When dispensing flea treatments you should advise that the owner treats the house/dog's bedding etc. and mention that the animal will need worming against tapeworm. This should all be recorded in the case log. You might also ask whether the client has any other animals that may need treating, e.g. cat.

7.5.2 Consistent with the Veterinary Surgeons' Act 1966, a veterinary surgeon must prescribe the medication being dispensed. The assessor may sign the log sheet with a statement in the assessor's comments confirming that the drugs dispensed have been prescribed by an identified veterinary surgeon and a statement confirming the student's competence at dispensing the drugs prescribed.

8 Guidance notes for modules 6–14

8.1 Laboratory and Diagnostic Aids – Section 6

It is important to show a wide range of cases that indicate that the student can perform various laboratory techniques.

A total of seven log sheets are required and, in addition, a copy of the results should be included ensuring the clients' details are omitted.

8.1.1 'Preparation of equipment':
Should take into account procedures such as allowing the biochemical machine to warm up or ensuring test slides are at room temperature before commencing the test.

8.1.2 'Preparation of sample for testing':
Although the procedure may be carried out immediately on the sample, it should still be noted whether the sample is to be mixed thoroughly or centrifuged.

8.1.3 'Procedure for test':
If a biochemical machine is used, then a *brief* explanation of the procedure may be included. It is not necessary, however, to go into detailed explanation of the workings of the biochemical analyser.

8.2 Fluid Management – Section 7

A total of three case logs is required which should include three of the range of fluids listed.

A fluid monitoring chart should also be included for each of the three case logs.

8.2.1   'Reason for administering fluid';
        Why fluid therapy was indicated this case.
8.2.2   'Type of fluid':
        Whether crystalloid or colloid etc.
8.2.3   'Reason for choice of fluid':
        This depends on what loss has occurred, i.e. primary water loss, electrolyte loss or blood loss.
8.2.5   'Route of administration':
        Intravenous is the fastest method but may not be applicable in exotics.
8.2.6   'Total volume to be given':
        Need to work out total requirements. This should include amount to rehydrate the animal, maintenance requirements and any ongoing losses.
8.2.7   'Reason why volume given':
        Show calculation of the above.
8.2.8   'Drip rate':
        If the fluid is administered iv, then drip rate should be calculated to 'drops per minute'. If a bolus is given, then this should be mentioned.
8.2.9   'Rate of administration':
        Calculate in ml/kg per hour. If there is an initial 'shock rate', i.e. a faster than normal rate is given for the first 1–2 hours, then this should also be mentioned.

8.2.10 'Urine output':
State how urine output was measured, i.e. urinary catheterisation or free catch.

8.3 Medical Nursing – Section 8

A total of eight case logs should be completed. Choose from a list or from the objective syllabus.

Three of the eight cases need to be in-depth, using the subheadings provided.

8.3.1 'Major presenting problem':
If this was not known when the animal was admitted, then it could be history from the owner, i.e. polydipsia, polyuria, lethargy etc.

8.3.2 'Principal clinical findings':
Findings from a clinical examination – temperature, pulse and respiration should be recorded as well as any abnormalities such as palpable superficial lymph nodes, enlarged abdomen, irregular or muffled heartbeat etc.

8.3.3 'Diagnostic tests':
Should include appropriate tests – blood analysis, urinalysis, radiography and ultrasonography etc. A brief explanation as to why these tests were carried out and what the results were should be included.

8.3.4 'Medical nursing':
Keep brief. Interesting cases can be expanded upon in a case report.

8.3.5 'Other nursing information':
How the case will be managed in the long term, information given to owners about treatment etc.

8.4 Radiography – Section 9

A total of ten cases that cover a broad spectrum of procedures. Try to cover a range of species in the case logs.

When choosing a case, concentrate on one area only that requires radiography. For example, if a case requires a pelvic radiograph as well as a chest radiograph, then it could be used for two case logs.

8.4.1 'Area to be radiographed':
For example, the abdomen.

8.4.2 'Patient preparation and restraint':
Whether general anaesthesia or sedation was used and whether sandbags, foam wedges and ties were used.

8.4.3 'Exposure factors':
The film focal distance should be expressed in metric units. With many machines, the kilo-voltage may be linked to the milliamperage setting. If this is the case, then mention it in the log sheet. The focal spot refers to whether the machine has fine focus or coarse focus. If it is not evident, then the phrase 'automatically adjusted' would suffice.

8.4.4 'View'
Radiograph projection, i.e. ventro-dorsal abdomen, caudo-cranial stifle.

8.4.5 'Positioning of the animal':
Should describe how the animal was positioned on the table, e.g. lateral recumbency with forelegs extended cranially.

8.4.6 'Centring details' and 'Collimation of primary beam':

Anatomical landmarks should be given to describe both centring and collimation.

8.4.7 'Appraisal of radiographical quality':
Is the radiograph of diagnostic quality or is it over- or under-exposed? Any extraneous marks? Is the area of interest in the centre of the radiograph or could the animal be positioned so that the area was in the centre?

8.4.8 'Health and safety issues':
Reference to Ionising Radiation Regulations and whether protective clothing was needed for a particular view.

8.5 Surgical Nursing – General – Section 10

Case logs
A total of ten logs in which three of the cases include a bandaging and dressing. Ensure the range of cases and species is covered.

Case reports
Three of the ten cases should be expanded into a case report, one of which should include a bandage and dressing.

It is important to concentrate on the nursing aspects of the case although you should have knowledge of the disease or condition.

Theatre practice – post-operative care
This case report could also be cross-referenced to a report from the case log/reports.

Notes

When completing the surgical nursing case logs, an appendix listing the instruments required may be more appropriate. If a general surgical kit is always used, then this could be an appendix and a list of additional instruments required listed in the case log.

Patient preparation including skin preparation may be similar in most cases and therefore this could be presented as an appendix and any alterations to the routine preparation could be listed.

8.6 Surgical Nursing – Theatre Practice – Section 11

Sterilization

Two log sheets, one using an autoclave and one using another method, i.e. hot air, oven, ethylene oxide, cold chemical etc.

Maintaining asepsis and sterility

A list of procedures carried out in theatre to maintain asepsis. This will include cleaning protocols and checking of sterilization procedures.

Pre-operative protocols may include damp dusting of theatres and ensuring all equipment needed is in the theatre to prevent too much moving about during operations.

During the operation – ensuring scrubbed personnel and sterile equipment is not contaminated.

Post-operatively – cleaning away any blood or bodily fluids and disposing of contaminated tissue. Cleaning the theatre before the next operation.

Maintaining equipment
Choose three items from the list and complete a log sheet.

Instruments
Produce a wall chart or poster with labelled illustrations of all instruments required by one of three procedures. Instrument catalogues may be a useful guide and reference source.

8.7 Anaesthesia – Section 12

A total of ten anaesthetic case logs which includes a range of species of animals.

Three of the ten cases must be in more detail, with at least one surgical case. For each of the three cases an anaesthetic record form should be included.

8.7.1　*The log sheet*
　　　　'Description of animal':
　　　　Whether the animal is overweight or thin, geriatric or very young.
　　　　'Risk category':
　　　　'Premedication and induction':
　　　　Dose rates should be in mg/kg or total dose in mg.

8.8 Other Species – Exotics – Section 13

A total of five cases is required with the addition of one more detailed case, using the same headings as the log sheet.

8.9 Health and Safety – Section 14

Three risk assessments on different areas of the practice.
'Description of activity':
For example, cleaning kennels, doing a blood smear, assisting with operations and preparation of an animal for surgery, taking radiographs, cleaning the waiting room floor.

9 Portfolio submission and outcomes

The RCVS issue guidelines for the submission of the veterinary nurse portfolio and these should always be confirmed prior to submission. At the time of publication the RCVS guidelines can be summarized as set out below.

Before submission of the relevant modules of the portfolio, special attention should be made to check the following:

- That all log sheets are completed in full and signed by both the SVN and assessor.
- That the authentication sheet in the portfolio lists all the signatures that appear in the portfolio with the designation of each individual being clearly documented.
- That all evidence that could identify a client by name, address or any other means recognizable outside the veterinary practice has been removed from the case logs and any supporting evidence.
- That all pages are numbered in the bottom right-hand corner and a contents list is enclosed at the front of the portfolio.
- That a hard copy of the entire submission is retained by the SVN. A copy on computer disk is inappropriate, as this will not have the relevant signatures and assessor comments.

The following items must be submitted for external verification:

- A submission form with the appropriate sections completed by the SVN and the practice principal.
- The personal profile and details of college-based training.
- The authentication sheet (fully completed).
- The action plan for the relevant level of S/NVQ.
- The case log sheets and any essential supporting evidence for the relevant modules.
- A contents list indexing all submitted papers.

If any of the above are omitted, the RCVS may return the portfolio as unsatisfactory and it will need to be submitted during the next examination period.

The following items should *not* be submitted:

- Portfolio folder.
- Log sheets for modules 6–14 (if submitting for the S/NVQ Level 2) or modules 1–5 (if submitting for S/NVQ Level 3).
- Module instructions.
- Commercially produced leaflets.
- Items that are not essential for the portfolio evidence.

9.1 Submission procedure

The submission sheets should be completed using BLACK INK and CAPITAL letters. The return address for the portfolio should be completed.

All the relevant items discussed above should be included and placed in the following order:

1 submissions sheet
2 contents list
3 personal profile sheets
4 authentication sheet
5 action plan
6 case log sheets

A copy of the entire submission should be kept.

Plastic wallets/pockets should *not* be submitted. Reinforcing rings should be used to strengthen the holes in any sheets where necessary.

The items above should be secured with treasury tags, placed in a strong envelope and posted to:

Royal College of Veterinary Surgeons
Belgravia House
62–64 Horseferry Road
London
SW1P 2AF

Recorded delivery is advised for posting and the SVN is advised to maintain the receipt as proof of posting until the portfolio is returned.

The portfolio may be delivered in person to Belgravia House between 9 a.m. and 4 p.m., Monday to Friday.

The RCVS considers the portfolio to remain the responsibility of the SVN until it reaches the RCVS and does not recommend any other means of delivery other than those stated above.

Five working days should be allowed for the portfolio to reach the RCVS and this should be taken into consideration when posting close to the submission deadline. Proof of posting is not considered sufficient evidence should the portfolio fail to meet the submission deadline. Any portfolio failing to meet the deadline is classified as failing to provide sufficient evidence and will need to be submitted during the following examination period.

9.2 Return of the portfolio

The RCVS aim to have the portfolio returned within six weeks following submission. During busy periods, for example near the submission deadline, they recognize that this may extend to eight weeks.

The returned portfolio also has the following accompanying documents:

- A copy of the submission form indicating whether or not the portfolio contains sufficient evidence to meet the national standards.
- A letter explaining the outcome and any action that may be necessary.
- A sealed envelope which contains a second copy of the EV's report which should be treated as confidential and given to the assessor. The assessor may then discuss any relevant issues with the SVN.

The practice principal is informed of the outcome of external verification and is sent the EV's report to highlight any action required by the assessor and IV.

10 Terminology

Although every effort has been made to make this publication as free of the 'jargon' that is commonly associated with S/NVQs as possible, it is necessary that all those involved with the S/NVQ are familiar with appropriate terminology. For clarity and ease of reference, a list of relevant terms and abbreviations is provided below.

Accreditation

The formal act by which the Qualification Curriculum Authority recognizes statements of competence and approves awarding bodies and their qualifications for inclusion in the NVQ framework.

Area of Competence

A subdivision of the total occupational field to which a set of NVQs relates.

Assessment

The process of collecting evidence and making judgements on whether performance criteria have been met.

Assessor	The person responsible for checking that the levels required for skills, knowledge and understanding have been achieved.
ATAC	Approved Training and Assessment Centre. Formerly known as an ATC, an Approved Training Centre. Veterinary practices that were approved as ATCs in the past by the RCVS will have to go through a re-approval process to train veterinary nurses towards the S/NVQs.
Award	A general term for that which is given to an individual for the attainment of an NVQ.
Awarding Body	The RCVS: a body approved by the Qualification Curriculum Authority for the purpose of awarding an NVQ.
Candidate	An individual undertaking an S/NVQ.
Certificate	A document issued to an individual by an awarding body, formally attesting to the attainment of an NVQ or a unit of competence.
Competence	The ability to perform in work roles or jobs to the standards required in employment.

Evidence Gatherer	A qualified veterinary surgeon or listed veterinary nurse who does not hold a TDLB qualification in assessment but may act as an assessor. All evidence assessed by an evidence gatherer is subject to assessment by a TDLB assessor and verification by an internal verifier.
External Verifier	Person appointed by the awarding body, the RCVS; they are responsible for checking and monitoring assessments carried out in ATACs.
Internal Verifier	Person who checks that the assessments are carried out fairly, consistently and to the standard required by the awarding body – in this case the RCVS.
Lead (or Standard Setting Body)	A body responsible for the specification of standards of competence, made up of representatives of employers, employees and professions, and their advisers, as appropriate.
Lead Body	The Veterinary Lead Body, who are responsible for the national standards for the veterinary nurse industry upon which the VN qualification is based.

Level	A subdivision of the NVQ framework used to define progressive degrees of competence.
NCVQ	National Council for Vocational Qualifications. A government body that has now been replaced by the QCA.
NVQ	National Vocational Qualification: the award based upon the occupational standards, offered in England, Wales and Northern Ireland.
NVQ Criteria	The principles with which qualifications and their awarding bodies must conform for their accreditation and recognition by the NCVQ.
NVQ Framework	The national system for ordering NVQs according to levels and areas of competence.
Occupation	The collective term for jobs in an area of employment which require common aspects of competence.
Occupational Standards	Details of which are in the RCVS *Training Centre Handbook*: 'guidelines to the practice to which students are assessed'.

Performance Criteria	The criteria which indicate the standard of performance required for the successful achievement of an element of competence.
QCA	Qualifications Curriculum Authority: the accrediting body for NVQs in England, Wales and Northern Ireland. The QCA is responsible for accrediting NVQs in all areas and for auditing every awarding body to check that appropriate systems are in place and are being implemented effectively.
RCVS	The Royal College of Veterinary Surgeons: the awarding body for the Veterinary Nursing S/NVQs.
SQA	Scottish Qualifications Authority: the accrediting body for SVQs in Scotland. The responsibilities of the SQA are similar to those of the QCA.
Standard (of performance)	The measure of performance required for the achievement of an element of competence as indicated by the related performance criteria.
Standard of Competence	The specification of competence for employment upon which an NVQ is based, stated in the form

	of title, units, elements and performance criteria.
SVN	A student veterinary nurse; also known as a *candidate* when working towards the Veterinary Nursing S/NVQ.
SVQ	Scottish Vocational Qualification: the award based upon the occupational standards, offered in Scotland.
TDLB	Training and Development Lead Body. The industry organization that has responsibility for the training and assessing awards.
Unit (of competence)	A primary subdivision of the competence required for the award of an NVQ, representing a discrete aspect of competence having meaning in employment which may be recognized and certificated independently as a credit towards an award. A unit is made up of elements of competence.

Appendix A: Example case log sheets for modules 1–5

CASE LOG SHEET: BASIC ANIMAL MANAGEMENT

Student Veterinary Nurse's Name:	VN Enrolment No.:
A NONYMOUS	1234

The evidence in this Log Sheet is a true representation of my involvement in the case described, and the work undertaken in compiling the log is my own.

Student Veterinary Nurse's Signature:

1. Case Number-Identification:

BAM 1 (SASHA)

2. Case Details:

Species: *CANINE*   Breed: *SHETLAND SHEEP DOG*

Sex: *FEMALE (ENTIRE)*   Age: *13 YEARS*   Weight: *10.8 KG*

3. Reason for Hospitalisation:

Hospitalised after surgical removal of an extensive mixed mammary tumour, left caudal abdominal gland

Reason for hospitalisation: In order to monitor the wound in the initial post-operative period and to allow the patient to recover completely from general anaesthesia

4. Type of Accommodation and Bedding Material used:

Kennel: *Width 60 cm   Depth 90 cm   Height 60 cm*

Construction: *Tiled breeze block walls, tiled floor, steel mesh door, locker-type kennel*

Bedding: *Newspaper and blanket*

5. Feeding Regime:

Initially, starvation with water given frequently in small quantities in the evening after surgery once she had returned to full consciousness.

On the morning following surgery, she received a small quantity (about 30 ml) of Waltham canine selected protein diet. She then had a further small meal, about ¼ can of canine selected protein, before being returned to her owner. This was given at approximately 1 p.m.

It is important to ensure adequate nutrition, especially protein intake, after surgery, in order to compensate for the increase in metabolic rate which takes place.

6. Grooming Regime and Nursing Care:

Post-operatively: the wound was gently cleaned to remove any trickles of blood around the surgical site. Any contamination of hairs around the shaved area was washed off. Observations of Sasha's vital signs were recorded.

The following day: her temperature and pulse were checked. The wound was checked again but required no cleaning. Her eyes, nose, anus and vulva were checked for discharge and her eyes were cleaned. Her coat was gently brushed to remove knots and tangles, using a pin brush.

7. Cleaning Protocol:

To include: type of disinfectant, – dilution of, mechanical cleaning procedures, frequency of cleaning etc.

After the bitch had stayed in overnight, her kennel had not been soiled. She was put in an outside run where she passed urine. Her blanket and paper were removed and the kennel brushed out to remove fluff/hair. A fresh blanket and fresh paper were then put in before she was brought back from the run.

After she had been discharged, the kennel was completely emptied. Moulting hair was brushed out. The whole kennel (floor, roof, walls and door) was scrubbed in Trigene, using a concentration of 1 part in 100 parts of warm water. It was then left empty until completely dry.

8. Date(s) of treatment:

To include: full time-scale range if appropriate

8/7/98 Admission and operation, then post-surgical hospitalisation overnight
9/7/98 Hospitalised until 3 p.m. when discharged to owner

Student's Comments:

To include: the part the student has played in this case

My role in this case was as a ward nurse in charge of all hospitalised cases that week (on our rota system). I was responsible for all aspects of care for this case as recorded in the above sections.

Sasha's recovery from surgery was uncomplicated. She had few problems associated with old age and her nursing care was, consequently, straightforward.

Assessor's Statement

The procedures and details associated with the basic animal management described, have been observed by me and have been carried out correctly and competently:

Comments:

Assessor's Name: **Date:**

Assessor's Qualifications:

Assessor's Signature:

LEAFLET FORMAT: COMMUNICATIONS

Student Veterinary Nurse's Name:	VN Enrolment No.:
A NONYMOUS	1234

The evidence in this Leaflet is my own work.

Student Veterinary Nurse's Signature:

1. Topic of Leaflet:

*POST-OPERATIVE CARE FOR ROUTINE OPERATIONS
(BITCH OVARIO-HYSTERECTOMY))*

2. Basic Information required by owner on subject:

Immediate: *Emphasise effects of general anaesthetic
Water on arrival home with no food for 3 hours, then small meals
Lead exercise only
Check wound three times daily, preventing interference from dog
Any concerns contact surgery*

Ongoing: *Stitches removed in 7 days (as not soluble)
Details about buster collar
Details about administering medication
Next appointment*

3. Possible Policies or Approaches:

All bitches are spayed at this practice, after their first season. On discharging they are given a post-operative care sheet.

However bitches can be spayed as early as 10 weeks, although there is a body of thought that this may prevent the bitch from fully maturing.

Soluble sutures can be used for closing the surgical wound therefore removing the need for the bitch to return to the practice for their removal.

The attached leaflet would be used to convey all the information to the owner. I have chosen an A4 presentation for clarity and ease of production. The style of presentation conforms with other literature used within the practice and would consequently complement the range. It can be produced within the surgery, keeping cost to a minimum whilst retaining flexibility.

4. Practice Policy (if appropriate):

All bitches are spayed after their first season.

Written and verbal instructions on post-operative care are given to owners on discharge.

Bitch returns for suture removal in 7 days (non-soluble sutures).

Student's Comments:

To include: details of how easy you found it to convey the advice verbally to the owner(s)

I discharged Emma, a three-year-old bitch, following her surgical procedure and gave advice accompanied with the post-operative care sheet to her owner.

I confirmed the owner's understanding and gave them the opportunity to ask questions regarding post-operative care.

This is a procedure with which I am familiar and carry out on a routine basis.

Assessor's Statement

The advice and information included in the Communications Leaflet has been conveyed to the client(s) by the student – this has been observed by me and I consider it to have been carried out both correctly and effectively:

Comments:

Assessor's Name: **Date:**

Assessor's Qualifications:

Assessor's Signature:

Any Vet
Veterinary Hospital
Somewhere
In the middle of
Nowhere
Tel: 01234 56789

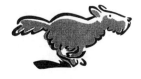

Post-operative Care Sheet

Name of Patient .... Date: ....

.... has had a general anaesthetic and may appear a little unsteady. S/He should be kept warm on returning home. After-effects of an anaesthetic may persist for a couple of days, although if you are concerned you should telephone us here at the hospital.

.... has had hair clipped from his/her leg where the anaesthetic has been injected.

Stitches are usually removed in 7 to 14 days. You will be advised when to return for this. You may have been given a buster collar to prevent .....
.... from interfering with the stitches.

Please follow the directions indicated below:

1. .... should be given water after arrival home. Food should be withheld for 3 hours, then small meals may be given.
2. The stitches are not soluble and need to be removed in .... days.
3. The surgical site should be inspected at reasonable intervals.
   .... may try to lick, bite or scratch the stitches, which should be prevented.
4. .... has been provided with a buster collar. This should be worn at all times except when s/he is eating, during which time s/he should be supervised.
5. .... should have lead exercise only for the first .... days.
6. Please give the tablets according to the instruction on the label.
7. .... needs to be seen again on ....

IF YOU ARE AT ALL CONCERNED ABOUT ....
CONDITION THEN PLEASE DO NOT HESITATE TO
CONTACT THE SURGERY.

CASE LOG SHEET: BASIC FIRST AID

Student Veterinary Nurse's Name:	VN Enrolment No.:
A NONYMOUS	*1234*

The evidence in this Log Sheet is a true representation of my involvement in the case described, and the work undertaken in compiling the log is my own.

Student Veterinary Nurse's Signature:

1. Case Number-Identification:

BFA 1 (BERT)

2. Case Details:

Species: *CANINE*   Breed: *JACK RUSSELL TERRIER*

Sex: *MALE (NEUTERED)*   *Age: 10 YEARS*   Weight: *9 KG*

3. History:

Deep incised wound sustained to right foreleg whilst out for exercise with owner.

4. Clinical evaluation of patient:

- *Moderate arterial haemorrhage from deep incision to palmar aspect of foreleg, proximal to metacarpal pad, approximately 4 cm in length*
- *Slightly ataxic but still standing*
- *Patient observed to be shivering and have cold peripheries*
- *Pale mucous membranes*
- *Capillary refill time – 2 seconds*
- *Tachypnoea/tachycardia*
- *Remained alert and responsive*

5. First Aid procedure carried out:

- *Owner arrives unexpectedly – no Veterinary Surgeon on premises.*
- *Patient wrapped in blanket to conserve body heat.*
- *Owner restrained patient.*
- *Sterile dressing (Melolin; Smith & Nephew) applied to wound and pressure bandage applied, enclosing whole foot and extending above the carpus until Veterinary Surgeon arrived.*

6. Student's Role:

- *Initial evaluation of patient*
- *Application of pressure bandage*
  - *sterile wound dressing covering wound*
  - *1 layer of cotton wool applied over whole foot*
  - *1 extra layer of cotton wool applied over wound*
  - *conforming bandage covering whole foot*
  - *white cohesive bandage applied as top bandage layer*
- *Contacted Veterinary Surgeon*
- *Observation of vital signs to ensure patient not deteriorating*
- *Observation of bandage to ensure no blood seeping through*

7. Outcome of First Aid:

- *No blood seen to soak through bandage therefore haemorrhage stemmed successfully*
- *Veterinary Surgeon arrived to provide further treatment*
- *Wound sutured under general anaesthesia*

8. Date(s):
To include: full time-scale range if appropriate

12.4.98   Patient admitted at 7.55 a.m.

Veterinary Surgeon arrived at 8.15 a.m.

Student's Comments:
To include: additional detail not given previously, and/or student's reflective comment

- *Patient discharged later same day*
- *I provided all initial first aid care and was pleased to see that application of the pressure bandage helped to stop the bleeding*

Assessor's Statement

The procedures and details associated with the Basic First Aid described, have been carried out correctly and competently by the student:

Comments:

Assessor's Name: **Date:**

Assessor's Qualifications:

Assessor's Signature:

CASE LOG SHEET: HUMAN FIRST AID

Student Veterinary Nurse's Name:	VN Enrolment No.:
A NONYMOUS	1234

The evidence in this Log Sheet is a true representation of my involvement in the case described, and the work undertaken in compiling the log is my own.

Student Veterinary Nurse's Signature:

1. Details of Occurrence:

Whilst holding a dog for examination my colleague, another Student Veterinary Nurse, was bitten on her right hand, drawing a small quantity of blood.

2. Details of Incident Book Entry:

Refer to attached photocopy of entry in accident report book.

3. First Aid procedure carried out:

- *The dog was removed to a kennel for temporary holding whilst first aid was administered*
- *After putting on protective gloves, I cleaned my colleague's wound under cold running water following which I applied dilute Savlon solution (1% dilution)*
- *I applied a clean, sterile swab to prevent further bleeding, applying slight pressure*
- *A plaster was applied to the wound as there was no further bleeding*
- *I advised my colleague to check the date of her last tetanus and to monitor the wound, seeking medical advice if it did not improve*

4. Student's role:

- *Removed dog to kennel*
- *Prepared and applied dilute (1%) Savlon solution, swab and plaster*
- *Recorded relevant details in accident report book*

5. Outcome:

My colleague was confident that the incident was minor and continued to restrain the dog (now muzzled) for further examination and treatment

6. Date(s):
To include: full time-scale range if appropriate

8/2/99 at approximately 10 a.m.

Student's Comments:

I administered the first aid myself under supervision of the Veterinary Surgeon (Mr A Vet MRCVS)

Witness Statement

NOTE: To be given when the incident has occurred outside the veterinary practice environment. It may be that your Assessor did not witness your involvement in such a case.

The procedures and details associated with the Human First Aid described, have been observed by me and have been carried out correctly and competently:

Signature: **Date:**

Name (print):

Assessor's Statement

NOTE: To be completed when the Assessor has been able to witness the incident and verify the student veterinary nurse's involvement.

The procedures and details associated with the Human First Aid described, have been observed by me and have been carried out correctly and competently:

Comments:

Assessor's Name: **Date:**

Assessor's Qualifications:

Assessor's Signature:

CASE LOG SHEET: DISPENSING RECORD

Student Veterinary Nurse's Name:	VN Enrolment No.:
A NONYMOUS	*1234*

The evidence in this Log Sheet is a true representation of my involvement in the case described, and the work undertaken in compiling the log is my own.

Student Veterinary Nurse's Signature:

1. Case Number-Identification:

DR 1

2. Case Details:

Species: *CANINE*   Breed: *LABRADOR RETRIEVER*

Sex: *MALE (ENTIRE)*   Age: *4½ YEARS*   Weight: *29 KG*

3. Name of drug dispensed (to include trade and generic names):

Trade name: Synulox

Generic name: Clavulanic acid potentiated amoxycillin

4. Dispensing Class and Prescribing Group:

Dispensing class: Prescription Only Medicine (POM)

Prescribing group: Antibiotic (broad spectrum)

5. Dose given (include calculations):

Dose rate:

12.5 mg per kg body weight, twice daily

Dose given (including calculation):

12.5 × 29 = 362.5 mg twice daily

Each tablet is 250 mg, therefore 362.5 mg/250 mg = 1.5 tablets twice daily

6. Reason for administration and route:

Broad spectrum antibiotic effective against bacteria causing pyoderma (deep bacterial skin infection)

Given orally as effective via this route and for ease of administration by client (palatable tablet)

7. Health & Safety, and other dispensing notes

To include: list of work products included, e.g. labels, controlled drug register entry copy, disposal of drugs (as appropriate)

- *Client instructed to give tablets at evenly spaced intervals (morning and night)*
- *Can be given with or without food, although palatable tablets so food should not be necessary*
- *Client instructed to wear gloves if hypersensitive to penicillins and to contact doctor if they have an adverse reaction to handling Synulox (see envelope attached)*

A printed label could be included here as evidence of the drug dispensed

8. Date(s) of treatment:

To include: full time-scale range if appropriate

8/2/99 to 18/2/99 inclusive

Student's Comments:

Although the envelope in which the tablets were dispensed detailed information regarding penicillin hypersensitivity, I drew the client's attention to this and discussed it with them so that I could be sure that they understood the information.

The client was asked to bring their dog back in 10 days (or sooner if the situation worsened or they had any other concerns)

Assessor's Statement

The procedures and details associated with the dispensing record described, have been observed by me and have been carried out correctly and competently:

Comments:

Assessor's Name: **Date:**

Assessor's Qualifications:

Assessor's Signature:

Appendix B: Example case log sheets for modules 6–14

CASE LOG SHEET: LABORATORY & DIAGNOSTIC AIDS

Student Veterinary Nurse's Name:	VN Enrolment No.:
A. Nonymous	1234

The evidence in this Log Sheet is a true representation of my involvement in the case described, and the work undertaken in compiling the log is my own.

Student Veterinary Nurse's Signature:

1. Case Number-Identification:

LAB 1

2. Case Details:

Species: CANINE   Breed: LABRADOR RETRIEVER

Sex: FEMALE (NEUTERED)   Age: 3 YEARS   Weight: 24 KG

3. Type of procedure and reasons for test:

Packed cell volume (PVC)/haematocrit to determine whether there was a significant increase which could help with assessing the degree of dehydration

4. Preparation of animal and pre-test procedures:

Skin turgor, colour of mucous membranes, capillary refill time (CRT) and urine specific gravity were all checked prior to blood sampling. The right forelimb was clipped to expose the cephalic vein and the site was cleansed with a dilute Hibiscrub solution, then surgical spirit was applied with a cotton wool swab. The patient was starved of food 12 hours prior to the procedure.

5. Equipment and supplies required:

Sterile 5 ml syringe + needle. Blood collection tube (EDTA: ethylene diamine tetra-acetic acid), gloves, dilute Hibiscrub/chlorhexidine, surgical spirit, cotton wool, clippers, microhaematocrit centrifuge/reader, plain capillary tubes, sealing compound: cristaseal, tissues.

6. Preparation of equipment:

The chlorhexidine solution was made fresh with warm water. The clippers were lubricated and the clipper blade checked to ensure no teeth were broken. The EDTA blood tubes were ready for immediate transfer of blood. The centrifuge was switched on, clean and ready for use.

7. Collection of sample:

The patient was lifted onto the table by the veterinary surgeon and myself. The dog was placed into sternal recumbency. I restrained the dog by placing my hand around its neck, holding the head away from the veterinary surgeon. Whilst holding behind the elbow of the right forelimb with the other hand, with my thumb I raised the vein. An additional person was needed to secure the animal's hindquarters. The veterinary surgeon performed venepuncture.

8. Preparation of sample for testing/storage and preservation, prior to dispatch:

The sample was immediately placed onto an EDTA blood tube, in which it was mixed gently by hand for 3–4 minutes using a rolling technique. The test was carried out immediately.

9. Procedure(s) for test or packaging and postage – method of dispatch:

A plain capillary tube was placed into the mixed blood until $\frac{3}{4}$ full. Holding horizontally, the tube was removed from the blood and wiped clean. Turning vertically the tube was placed into the sealing compound using both hands to twist and plug one end. The sealed tube was then transferred into the microhaematocrit centrifuge @ 1000 rpm for 5 min.

10. Results of test:

The result was determined by the use of a microhaematocrit reader.

Result = 45%

11. Normal Ranges:

Canine: 37–57%

12. Examples of conditions which may cause abnormal results:

Increase: dehydration

Decrease: anaemia/haemorrhage

13. Possible reasons for inaccurate results:

Sample insufficiently mixed, delay in testing sample, coagulation

14. Date(s):

To include: full time-scale of range if appropriate

Student's Comments:

It must be remembered that dehydration/anaemia cannot be diagnosed solely on a PCV result if the patient's PCV was not known previously, and that two samples should always be tested to ensure reliability of the procedure/technique.

Assessor's Statement

The procedures and details associated with the test described have been observed by me and have been carried out correctly and competently:

Comments:

Assessor's Name: **Date:**

Assessor's Qualifications:

Assessor's Signature:

CASE LOG SHEET: LABORATORY & DIAGNOSTIC AIDS

Student Veterinary Nurse's Name:	VN Enrolment No.:
A. Nonymous	1234

The evidence in this Log Sheet is a true representation of my involvement in the case described, and the work undertaken in compiling the log is my own.

Student Veterinary Nurse's Signature:

1. Case Number-Identification:

LAB 2

2. Case Details:

Species: FELINE   Breed: DSH DOMESTIC SHORT HAIR
Sex: MALE (ENTIRE)   Age: 7 MONTHS   Weight: 3 KG

3. Type of procedure and reasons for test:

Urinalysis: recurring cystitis cystocentesis

4. Preparation of animal and pre-test procedures:

The animal's temperature, pulse and respiration were checked along with capillary refill time, colour of mucous membranes and skin turgor. Food had been withdrawn for 12 hours, and the bladder was palpated to ensure it wasn't empty or too full to perform the procedure. A 5 × 5 cm area was clipped on the midline caudal abdomen and cleaned aseptically with chlorhexidine.

5. Equipment and supplies required:

Clippers, gloves, dilute chlorhexidine solution and surgical spirit. Sterile 10 ml syringe + 23 gauge × 1" needle. Urine collection pots: boric acid/plain, urine reagent, dipsticks, pipettes, centrifuge + tubes, microscope slides, coverslip, mounting needle.

6. Preparation of equipment:

Urinary dipsticks were checked to ensure they had not been damaged or contaminated in any way and that they were within the expiry date. The chlorhexidine solution was made fresh with warm H_2O. The clippers were lubricated and the blade checked for broken teeth. The centrifuge was switched on ready for use.

7. Collection of sample:

The patient was restrained by myself in left and lateral recumbency, with hind limbs extended caudally. The veterinary surgeon manually immobilised the bladder through the abdominal wall. The needle was then inserted through the abdominal wall into the bladder and urine was then withdrawn into the syringe. Once the needle was removed I replaced digital pressure at the injection site.

8. Preparation of sample for testing/storage and preservation prior to dispatch:

The urine was equally divided into a plain universal container and boric acid container and the tests were immediately carried out.

9. Procedure(s) for test or packaging and postage – method of dispatch:

A drop of urine was placed on each reagent strip on the urinary dipstick and read against the colour chart at the appropriate times. Urine was transferred to $\frac{3}{4}$ fill two centrifuge tubes and the samples were spun for 4 minutes @ 400 rpm using a microhaematocrit centrifuge. The supernatant fluid was removed using a sterile pipette and the sediment was then transferred onto a microscope slide and a coverslip applied. It was then examined under a microscope.

10. Results of test:

pH 7.0   Ketones negative   Specific gravity 1.008
Blood +++   Glucose negative   Microscopy: triple phosphate crystals seen
Protein ++   Urobilinogen negative

11. Normal Ranges:

pH 6–7   Specific gravity 1.020–1.040

A little protein + urobilinogen can be normal, everything else should appear negative

12. Examples of conditions which may cause abnormal results:

1. Blood: cystitis, neoplasia, nephritis
2. Specific gravity (decrease): pyometra, diabetes insipidus, increased H_2O intake
3. Protein: haematuria, pyuria, cystitis
4. Struvite/triple phosphate crystals: staphylococcal infections, alkaline urine

13. Possible reasons for inaccurate results:

Reading results at the wrong time; dipsticks out of date; alkaline urine can affect protein result; prolonged storage.

14. Date(s):

To include: full time-scale of range if appropriate

Student's Comments:

Urine must be tested immediately when at all possible or preserved. Cystocentesis is the preferred method for obtaining urine for urinalysis as, if carried out correctly, it is the most sterile method.

Assessor's Statement

The procedures and details associated with the test described have been observed by me and have been carried out correctly and competently:

Comments:

Assessor's Name: Date:

Assessor's Qualifications:

Assessor's Signature:

CASE LOG SHEET: FLUID MANAGEMENT

Student Veterinary Nurse's Name:	VN Enrolment No.:

The evidence in this Log Sheet is a true representation of my involvement in the case described, and the work undertaken in compiling the log is my own.
Student Veterinary Nurse's Signature:

1. Case Number-Identification:

A1

2. Case Details:

Species: FELINE   Breed: PERSIAN

Sex: FEMALE (ENTIRE)   Age: 9 YEARS   Weight: KG

3. Reason for Administering Fluid:

Anorexic

4. Type of Fluid given:

Hartmann's

5. Reason for choice of Fluid:

Hartmann's is a balanced electrolyte solution suitable for replacing primary losses

6. Route of Administration, and why route was selected:

Intravenous into cephalic vein – most effective method of replacing losses

7. Total Volume to be given:

Maintenance requirements: 50 ml/kg per 24 hr = 20 ml

5% dehydration: (5/100) × 4 = 0.2 litres (200 ml)

Total = 400 ml over 24 hr

8. Reason why Volume was given:

The cat requires maintenance, as it is still not eating. Also need to take into account continuing losses.

9. Drip rate (if appropriate):

400 ml over 24 hr   Burette delivers 60 drops/ml

= 16.7 ml/hr

= 0.3 ml/min

= 17 drops/min

10. Rate of Administration:

4 ml/kg per hr

11. Urine Output:

The volume of urine was not measured accurately but the cat passed a small amount during the afternoon

12. Date(s):

To include: full time-scale range if appropriate

3/6/98 Cat admitted for fluid therapy

4/6/98 Cat discharged

Student's Comments:

I was responsible for the care of the cat throughout the hospitalisation period. I completed all documentation associated with the fluid administration.

Assessor's Statement

The procedures and details associated with the fluid management described have been observed by me and have been carried out correctly and competently:

Comments:

Assessor's Name: **Date:**

Assessor's Qualifications:

Assessor's Signature:

CASE LOG SHEET: FLUID MANAGEMENT

Student Veterinary Nurse's Name:	VN Enrolment No.:

The evidence in this Log Sheet is a true representation of my involvement in the case described, and the work undertaken in compiling the log is my own.

Student Veterinary Nurse's Signature:

1. Case Number-Identification:

A2

2. Case Details:

Species: CANINE   Breed: LABRADOR

Sex: MALE   Age: 3 YEARS   Weight: 30 KG

3. Reason for Administering Fluid:

Surgery to repair a fractured femur; fluid therapy is given to replace primary water loss.

4. Type of Fluid given:

Dextrose + 4% saline 0.18%

5. Reason for choice of Fluid:

Isotonic solution for general maintenance

6. Route of Administration, and why route was selected:

The fluid was administered intravenously via the cephalic vein. This is the most efficient and quickest method of giving fluid.

7. Total Volume to be given:

Surgical maintenance is $5 \times$ maintenance $= 5 \times 50$ ml/kg per 24 hr

$$= 250\,\text{ml} \times 30$$

$$= 7500\,\text{ml over 24 hr}$$

8. Reason why Volume was given:

During surgery primary water loss may occur via evaporation from tissues. Anaesthesia incurs water loss from breathing cold gases.

Surgery may incur blood loss – excessive blood loss would be corrected by giving whole blood or colloids.

9. Drip rate (if appropriate):

7500 ml per 24 hr   A standard giving set delivers 20 drops/ml

= 312.5 ml/hr

= 5.2 ml/min

= 104 drops/min

~ 2 drops/sec

10. Rate of Administration:

Rate of 250 ml/kg per 24 hr

11. Urine Output:

The dog was catheterized before surgery. The urinary catheter was then attached to a collecting bag. The dog had produced 100 ml by the end of the surgery.

12. Date(s):
To include: full time-scale range if appropriate

11/11/99 Dog admitted.

12/11/99 Radiographs taken before surgery. Fluids removed 4 hours after surgery.

13/11/99 Dog discharged.

Student's Comments:

I was involved with the restraint and supervision of the dog during the administration of its fluids.

Assessor's Statement

The procedures and details associated with the fluid management described have been observed by me and have been carried out correctly and competently:

Comments:

Assessor's Name: **Date:**

Assessor's Qualifications:

Assessor's Signature:

CASE LOG SHEET: MEDICAL NURSING

Student Veterinary Nurse's Name:	VN Enrolment No.:

The evidence in this Log Sheet is a true representation of my involvement in the case described, and the work undertaken in compiling the log is my own.

Student Veterinary Nurse's Signature:

1. Case Number-Identification:

MN1

2. Case Details:

Species: FELINE   Breed: D.S.H.

Sex: MALE (NEUTERED)   Age: 5 YEARS   Weight: 3.5 KG

3. Major presenting problem:

Anorexia, weight loss – gradual onset over last 4 weeks

4. Principal clinical findings:

Temperature, pulse and respiration were within normal limits. Weight loss and slight tenting of the skin indicating dehydration.

5. Diagnostic tests, results & significance of tests carried out:

PCV was within normal limits. Biochemistry shows an increase in blood urea nitrogen and creatinine levels indicating a renal problem.

6. Medical Nursing

To include: medication, fluid therapy, dietary management & general nursing

Fluid therapy was initiated at a rate of 7 ml/kg per hr. Hartmann's was used as a balanced electrolyte solution. As the cat had not been eating it was offered chicken and a small amount of warmed A/D. The cat was not keen to eat at first and so was maintained on fluid therapy. However, overnight, the cat ate a small amount of chicken. The fluid therapy was maintained but at a rate of 4 ml per kg per hr throughout the next day, although the cat was now eating small amounts of low protein diet.

The blood biochemistry was rechecked the following day and the levels of BUN and creatinine had decreased to almost within normal limits.

The cat was now eating well and so fluid therapy was stopped. Antibiotics were started when the cat was admitted and continued for a further 7 days.

7. Other Nursing Information

To include: long-term management & information for clients

With patients that are suffering from renal failure it is important to feed a low protein diet. However, if an animal has been anorexic it is equally important to ensure the animal starts eating again. Chicken is high in good-quality protein but very palatable. The cat was discharged with a low protein diet. Blood tests were taken after 1 week to check the biochemistry levels – they were within normal limits.

8. Date(s):

To include: full time-scale range if appropriate

29/10/99 Cat admitted for blood test and fluid therapy

1/11/99 Cat discharged with medication and special low protein diet

Student's Comments:

In this case it was important to ensure that the cat was eating. Chicken was offered as it is very palatable, although high in protein. The fluid therapy made the cat feel better which also helped to retain its appetite.

Assessor's Statement

The procedures and details associated with the Medical Nursing described have been observed by me and have been carried out correctly and competently:

Comments:

Assessor's Name: **Date:**

Assessor's Qualifications:

Assessor's Signature:

CASE LOG SHEET: RADIOGRAPHY

Student Veterinary Nurse's Name:	VN Enrolment No.:

The evidence in this Log Sheet is a true representation of my involvement in the case described, and the work undertaken in compiling the log is my own.

Student Veterinary Nurse's Signature:

1. Case Number-Identification:

R1

2. Case Details:

Species: CANINE   Breed: GERMAN SHEPHERD

Sex: MALE (ENTIRE)   Age: 3 YEARS   Weight: 43 KG

3. Area to be radiographed:

Pelvis

4. Patient preparation and restraint:

Sedation with 2 mg acepromazine maleate (ACP: BK.ACE) subcutaneously

Anaesthesia with 250 mg thiopentone 2.5% intravenously

Calving ropes and a trough were used

5. Recording equipment:

Screen Type: Trimax T8   Film Type: Trimax 3m   Grid: Potter Bucky

6. Exposure Factors:

FFD: 37 inches   kV: 85   mAs: 25   Focal spot size/area: Automatically adjusted

7. View, e.g. ventral, dorsal:

1. Ventro-dorsal (VD)
2. Lateral (Right) (Rlat)

8. Positioning of Animal

1. Animal placed in trough and calving ropes used for parallel positioning of femoral
2. R. lat animal positioned using foam wedges and calving ropes

9. Centring details:

1. VD centred on pubic symphysis
2. R. lat centred on left greater trochanter

10. Collimation of primary beam:

1. Cranially iliac crests; caudally proximal tibias; laterally lateral borders of torso.
2. Cranially iliac crests; caudally – perineum, dorsal border of torso ventral mid-shaft femur.

11. Appraisal of radiographical quality:

There was a slight tilt to the right on the ventro-dorsal view. Centring and collimation were good on the lateral view, although the proximal and caudal edges were not contained within the border of the film on the VD view and therefore collimation is poor on this view. The film was slightly over-exposed but bony detail was good. There were some dust specks on the film from dirty intensifying screens.

12. Health and Safety Issues:

Related to bone comments.

1. Poor collimation means that area of primary beam is not known.
2. Film slightly over-exposed, which means that the kV was too high increasing the risk of scatter.

General H&S issues include those concerned with the Ionising Regulations 1985 + Approved Code of Practice for the protection of persons against ionising radiation arising from any work activity. Manual Handling Operations Legislation 1992

13. Veterinary Surgeon's diagnosis:

Severely arthritic hip (L)

Recommend hip replacement

14. Date(s):

To include: full time-scale range if appropriate

13/8/99 Admitted for general anaesthesia and radiography; the dog was discharged later that day.

Student's Comments:

I would ensure that the collimation was within the borders of the x-ray plate. Reduce the kV for the next dog of the same size having the same study. Ensure correct positioning with no rotation/tilting of the VD view.

Assessor's Statement

The procedures and details associated with the radiographic record described, have been observed by me and have been carried out correctly and competently:

Comments:

Assessor's Name: **Date:**

Assessor's Qualifications:

Assessor's Signature:

CASE LOG SHEET: RADIOGRAPHY

Student Veterinary Nurse's Name:	VN Enrolment No.:

The evidence in this Log Sheet is a true representation of my involvement in the case described, and the work undertaken in compiling the log is my own.

Student Veterinary Nurse's Signature:

1. Case Number-Identification:

R2

2. Case Details:

Species: CANINE   Breed: WEST HIGHLAND WHITE TERRIER

Sex: MALE (ENTIRE)   Age: 6 MONTHS   Weight: 5 KG

3. Area to be radiographed:

Skull

4. Patient preparation and restraint:

Sedation with 0.5 mg acepromazine maleate (ACP: BK.ACE) subcutaneously

Anaesthesia with propofol 25 mg (Rapinovet)

Sandbags were used for restraint of the head for the skull radiographs

5. Recording equipment:

Screen Type: Orthofine Green seal Film Type: Green seal (Ciba Geigy) Grid: N/A

6. Exposure Factors:

FFD: 37 inches   kV: 62   mAs: 15   Focal spot size/area: Automatically adjusted

7. View, e,g, ventral, dorsal:

1. Dorso-ventral view
2. Lateral

8. Positioning of Animal

1. Dog was placed in sternal recumbency with the neck extended; a sandbag was placed over the neck.
2. Dog was placed in lateral recumbency. The nose and mandible were raised so that the skull was parallel with plate.

9. Centring details:

1. Beam was centred between the eyes.
2. Beam was centred midway between the eye and the ear.

10. Collimation of primary beam:

1. Cranially/rostrally: tip of nose Caudally: C1/C2 Laterally: lateral borders of head
2. Rostrally: tip of nose Caudally: C1 Laterally: lateral borders of head

11. Appraisal of radiographical quality:

The dorso-ventral view of the skull was not straight, therefore the whole image was rotated. Otherwise good collimation and centring was fine on the lateral view, as was the collimation. The film was developed by automatic processor and the quality was good. There were some extraneous marks caused by dirt on the intensifying screen. There were some fingerprints on film made after processing.

12. Health and Safety Issues:

None related to above comments.

General H&S issues include those concerned with the Ionising Regulations 1985 + Approved Code of Practice for the protection of persons against ionising radiation arising from any work activity. Health & Safety at Work Act 1974. Manual Handling Operations Legislation 1992.

13. Veterinary Surgeon's diagnosis:

Cranial-mandibular osteopathy

14. Date(s):

To include: full time-scale range if appropriate

8/11/99 The dog was admitted for radiography and discharged the same day.

Student's Comments:

This was quite a difficult area to radiograph and I tried to get the skull straight on a couple of occasions.

Assessor's Statement

The procedures and details associated with the radiographic record described, have been observed by me and have been carried out correctly and competently:

Comments:

Assessor's Name: **Date:**

Assessor's Qualifications:

Assessor's Signature:

CASE LOG SHEET: RADIOGRAPHY

Student Veterinary Nurse's Name:	VN Enrolment No.:

The evidence in this Log Sheet is a true representation of my involvement in the case described, and the work undertaken in compiling the log is my own.

Student Veterinary Nurse's Signature:

1. Case Number-Identification:

R3

2. Case Details:

Species: CANINE   Breed: ROTTWEILER

Sex: MALE (ENTIRE)   Age: 6 YEARS   Weight: 39.5 KG

3. Area to be radiographed:

Right stifle

4. Patient preparation and restraint:

The dog was premedicated with acepromazine, butorphanol and atropine. It was then anaesthetised with thiopentone.

Sandbags and ties were then used to position the dog.

5. Recording equipment:

Screen Type: Rare Earth   Film Type: Fuji HRG   Grid: No grid used

6. Exposure Factors:

FFD: 102 cm   kV: 55   mAs: 3 (100 × 0.03)   Focal spot size/area: Fine focus

7. View, e.g. ventral, dorsal:

Lateral stifle

8. Positioning of animal

The dog was placed in lateral recumbency. The left leg was abducted and secured with ties.

9. Centring details:

1. Beam was centred on the distal femoral condyle.

10. Collimation of primary beam:

The beam was collimated to include the proximal 1/3 of the tibia and the distal 1/3 of the femur.

11. Appraisal of radiographical quality:

Good positioning, although there was slight rotation on the lateral stifle. The film was processed automatically.

12. Health and Safety Issues:

Ionising Regulations 1985

Health & Safety at Work Act 1974

COSHH Regulations 1988

Local Radiation Regulations

13. Veterinary Surgeon's diagnosis:

Ruptured cruciate ligament in the right stifle

14. Date(s):

To include: full time-scale range if appropriate

23/8/99 Dog admitted for radiography and subsequently operated on to repair the rupture.

24/8/99 Discharged.

Student's Comments:

Radiographs were taken of both stifles – lateral and cranio-caudal views were taken for comparison.

Assessor's Statement

The procedures and details associated with the radiographic record described, have been observed by me and have been carried out correctly and competently:

Comments:

Assessor's Name: **Date:**

Assessor's Qualifications:

Assessor's Signature:

CASE LOG SHEET: SURGICAL NURSING – GENERAL

Student Veterinary Nurse's Name:	VN Enrolment No.:

The evidence in this Log Sheet is a true representation of my involvement in the case described, and the work undertaken in compiling the log is my own.

Student Veterinary Nurse's Signature:

1. Case Number-Identification:

STRMF

2. Case Details:

Species: FELINE   Breed: DSH

Sex: MALE (NEUTERED)   Age: ADULT   Weight: 4.1 KG

3. Major presenting problems:

Fractured right hind limb – 4 weeks old (approx.)

4. Reason(s) for surgery:

To amputate hind limb as surgical repair was considered infeasible.

5. Diagnostic tests, results & significance of tests used:

X-rays of limb, lateral and caudo–cranial.

These were taken to confirm that no healing had taken place and that the fracture was beyond repair, and that no further injuries or underlying disease existed. He was also blood tested for FIV/FELV.

6. Surgical Nursing

To include: patient preparation, fluid therapy, analgesia, anaesthesia used (if appropriate), instrumentation required and general nursing

- The cat was premedicated 20 minutes before surgery with acepromazine and buprenorphine.
- Induction was with alphaxalone and alphadalone and maintained on isoflurane.
- When anaesthetised the limb was clipped and then cleaned and prepared with a chlorhexidine 4% solution.
- He was not given any intravenous fluid therapy.
- Analgesia was included in the premedication.
- The surgical kit used was a standard pack with no special instruments needed.

7. Other Nursing Information

To include: post-operative care & aftercare (which might include hospitalisation, bandaging, pain management, medication etc.), long-term management & information for clients

- The cat was a stray and stayed in hospital post-operatively until a home was found for him.
- He was given post-operative buprenorphine for the 24 hours following the operation.
- He was put on a 5-day course of antibiotics which were given orally in food to avoid the extra stress of injections.
- An Elizabethan collar was placed on the cat as he tried to remove his stitches.

8. Post-operative complications:

Several of the sutures had been placed quite tightly and caused the cat discomfort, both while they were in place and on removal.

9. Date(s):

To include: full time-scale range if appropriate

16/11/99–20/11/99

Student's Comments:

This cat was a great favourite due to his long stay in hospital and my close involvement with his care as the nurse in charge of his case. The cat recovered quickly and was soon mobile.

Assessor's Statement

The procedures and details associated with the Surgical Nursing described, have been observed by me and have been carried out correctly and competently:

Comments:

Assessor's Name: **Date:**

Assessor's Qualifications:

Assessor's Signature:

CASE LOG SHEET: SURGICAL NURSING – GENERAL

Student Veterinary Nurse's Name:	VN Enrolment No.:

The evidence in this Log Sheet is a true representation of my involvement in the case described, and the work undertaken in compiling the log is my own.

Student Veterinary Nurse's Signature:

1. Case Number-Identification:

STE14

2. Case Details:

Species: IGUANA   Breed: GREEN

Sex: FEMALE   Age: 3 YEARS   Weight: 2.8 KG

3. Major presenting problems:

Egg-bound

4. Reason(s) for surgery:

Ovariohysterectomy – to remove uterus and ovaries

5. Diagnostic tests, results & significance of tests used:

Radiography – to confirm diagnosis on presenting signs

Ventro-dorsal abdomen showed egg-bound uterus

6. Surgical Nursing

To include: patient preparation, fluid therapy, analgesia, anaesthesia used (if appropriate), instrumentation required and general nursing

- Prior to surgery the iguana was not starved but an intra-osseous catheter was introduced into the left femur and the iguana was maintained on Hartmann's at 24 ml/kg per 24 hr.
- The surgical site was prepared with povidone-iodine scrub.
- Analgesia was given although its efficacy is unknown – carprofen 4 mg/kg and buprenorphine 0.1 mg/kg.
- A fine surgical kit was used including Metzenbaum scissors and ophthalmic forceps.
- The operating theatre was kept at a temperature of 30°C to maintain the poikilotherm's temperature.
- Anaesthesia was induced by ketamine injection and maintained on isoflurane.

7. Other Nursing Information

To include: post-operative care & aftercare (which might include hospitalisation, bandaging, pain management, medication etc.), long-term management & information for clients

- Post-operatively it was very important to maintain body temperature and fluid levels; the environmental temperature was measured regularly.
- The iguana was tube-fed a meal of cat food post-operatively until it was interested in food
- Antibiotics were given post-operatively (enrofloxacin) by subcutaneous injection; it is important to give injections between scales to prevent damage to the skin.
- Polyglactin 910 sutures were placed in the skin as these are absorbable and prevent the need to stress the animal further in order to remove sutures at a later date.

8. Post-operative complications (if appropriate):

The iguana recovered well and soon started to eat.

9. Date(s):

To include: full time-scale range if appropriate

21/1/00–23/1/00

Student's Comments:

I was involved in this case both in preparing the iguana for surgery and also in its aftercare, until it was ready to go home.

Assessor's Statement

The procedures and details associated with the Surgical Nursing described, have been observed by me and have been carried out correctly and competently:

Comments:

Assessor's Name: **Date:**

Assessor's Qualifications:

Assessor's Signature:

LOG SHEET: STERILISATION USING AN AUTOCLAVE

Student Veterinary Nurse's Name:	VN Enrolment No.:

The evidence in this Log Sheet is a true representation of my involvement in the case described, and the work undertaken in compiling the log is my own.

Student Veterinary Nurse's Signature:

1. Describe the type of autoclave used at your practice:

(Note: If no autoclave at your practice provide details of the autoclave on which you have gained experience and on which you have been assessed)

Model: Little Sister (Ellman)   Type: Vacuum Assisted

2. List the equipment and supplies that may be sterilised by autoclave:

- Instruments
- Gowns and drapes
- Swabs

3. State the materials which you use for packaging:

D.R.G. paper and polythene 'peel 'n' seal bags' of different sizes

4. For TWO different types of materials and equipment, give the exact procedure for operating the autoclave:

a. Name of material: Osteotome

Procedure:

The end of the osteotome is wrapped in a swab to stop the instrument damaging the bag. It is placed in an autoclave bag and after the air has been removed it is sealed.

Working pressure: 15 p.s.i.   Temperature: 121°C   Sterilising time: 15 min

b. Name of material: Gowns

Procedure:

The gown is folded correctly and placed in a corrugated autoclave box and sealed with Bowie Dick tape.

Working pressure: 15 p.s.i.   Temperature: 121°C   Sterilising time: 15 min

5. Give examples of why sterilisation may be inefficient:

- Incorrect use of autoclave
- Instrument not clean
- Packaging damaged

6. Give two other methods of sterilisation that can be used for the same equipment as in Item 2 above:

Ethylene oxide

Gamma irradiation

7. State two advantages and two disadvantages of sterilisation by using an autoclave:

Advantages:

● Quick method
● Can be used for wide range of equipment

Disadvantages:

● If no drying cycle, then items can be still wet
● Plastic items may melt using this method

Student's Comments:

In the practice we also have access to ethylene oxide – so we can sterilise plastics and fibre-optic equipment.

Assessor's Statement

The equipment and procedures described are reflective of those at this training and assessment centre. The student veterinary nurse is competent to carry out these sterilisation procedures to the required national standard:

Comments:

Assessor's Name: **Date:**

Assessor's Qualifications:

Assessor's Signature:

LOG SHEET: STERILISATION USING AN AUTOCLAVE

Student Veterinary Nurse's Name:	VN Enrolment No.:

The evidence in this Log Sheet is a true representation of my own work.

Student Veterinary Nurse's Signature:

1. Describe the type of autoclave used at your practice:

(Note: If no autoclave at your practice provide details of the autoclave on which you gained experience and on which you have been assessed)

Model: Little Sister   Type: Vacuum assisted

2. List the equipment and supplies that may be sterilised by autoclave:

Drapes, gowns, swabs, some plastic and rubber articles, stainless steel instruments

3. State the materials which you use for packaging:

Nylon film, Bowie Dick tape, water repellent paper and linen

4. For TWO different types of materials and equipment, give the exact procedure for operating the autoclave:

a. Name of material: Surgical gown

Procedure:

The gown was loaded onto the top tray, the water port was checked and filled up, the interior chamber was then filled by depressing the water fill button to cover the filaments, the door was securely closed and the start button depressed to commence the cycle.

Working pressure: 30 p.s.i.   Temperature: 134°C   Sterilising time: $3\frac{1}{2}$ minutes

b. Name of equipment: Bone cutters

Procedure:

As above.

Working pressure: Temperature: Sterilising time:

5. Give examples of why sterilisation may be inefficient:

- Overloading autoclave
- Incorrect packaging
- Incorrect cycle
- Instruments incorrectly cleaned, presence of grease, organic matter etc.

6. Give two other methods of sterilisation that can be used for the same equipment as in Item 2 above:

Ethylene oxide (anprolene): for various rubber, plastic and fibre-optic equipment

Hot air oven: for glassware and delicate cutting instruments

7. State two advantages and two disadvantages of sterilisation by using an autoclave:

Advantages:

- Process is quick
- Wide range of equipment can be sterilised by this method

Disadvantages:

- Human error
- Cannot sterilise electrical equipment

Student's Comments:

We use the vacuum-assisted autoclave for all our equipment although we do have access to ethylene oxide at our local hospital.

Assessor's Statement

The equipment and procedures described are reflective of those at this training and assessment centre. The student veterinary nurse is competent to carry out these sterilisation procedures to the required national standard:

Comments:

Assessor's Name: **Date:**

Assessor's Qualifications:

Assessor's Signature:

LOG SHEET: STERILISATION (OTHER THAN BY USING AN AUTOCLAVE)

Student Veterinary Nurse's Name:	VN Enrolment No.:

The evidence in this Log Sheet is a true representation of my own work.

Student Veterinary Nurse's Signature:

1. State the method of sterilisation:

Hot Air Oven

2. Describe the equipment used to carry out this sterilisation:

To include: details of model, type if appropriate

Model: Eschman Hot Air Oven   Type: Fan Assisted Oven

3. Describe any other supplies used to carry out this sterilisation:

Trays for the instruments to be placed on.

4. State what articles are sterilised by this method:

- Instruments – especially fine cutting instruments
- Glassware
- Powders

5. Describe the procedure for sterilisation using this equipment:

To include: working pressure, temperature and sterilising times (if appropriate)

The instruments are carefully cleaned, dried and lubricated. Any excess lubricant is removed. The instruments are laid on the trays and put in the oven.

Working pressure: N/A   Temperature: 150°C   Sterilising time: 180 minutes

6. State any advantages, disadvantages and discuss the limitations, if any, of this method of sterilisation:

Advantages:

● Doesn't dull cutting edges
● Easy to use

Disadvantages:

● Long time to complete cycle
● Cannot use for drapes/gowns

Student's Comments:

One of the main disadvantages is the length of time to complete cycle – sterilisation time does not include warm-up or cool-down period.

Assessor's Statement

The equipment and procedures described are reflective of those at this training and assessment centre. The student veterinary nurse is competent to carry out these sterilisation procedures to the required national standard:

Comments:

Assessor's Name: **Date:**

Assessor's Qualifications:

Assessor's Signature:

LOG SHEET: STERILISATION (OTHER THAN BY USING
AN AUTOCLAVE)

Student Veterinary Nurse's Name:	VN Enrolment No.:

The evidence in this Log Sheet is a true representation of my own work.
Student Veterinary Nurse's Signature:

1. State the method of sterilisation:

Ethylene oxide

2. Describe the equipment used to carry out this sterilisation:
To include: details of model, type if appropriate

Model: AN74V   Type: Anprolene Sterilizer

3. Describe any other supplies used to carry out this sterilisation:

Anprolene vial

Gas release bag

4. State what articles are sterilised by this method:

● Endoscopes
● Plastics (e.g. syringes, drains)
● Fibre-optics
● Rubber (E/T tubes)

5. Describe the procedure for sterilisation using this equipment:

To include: working pressure, temperature and sterilising times (if appropriate)

12 hours sterilising

12–24 hours airing

Working pressure: Temperature: Sterilising time:

6. State any advantages, disadvantages and discuss the limitations, if any, of this method of sterilisation:

Advantages:

- Plastics, fibre-optics, suture materials etc. cannot be done in autoclave
- Inactivates DNA, preventing cell reproduction, and therefore destroys bacteria and viruses

Disadvantages:

- Highly toxic, irritant, flammable gas, poisonous, cytotoxic
- Time consuming

Student's Comments:

Ethylene oxide is potentially very harmful, so safety issues must be adhered to.

Assessor's Statement:

The practice does not routinely use ethylene oxide as a method of sterilisation; however the student veterinary nurse is familiar with the procedures and health and safety implications of this agent.

Comments:

Assessor's Name: **Date:**

Assessor's Qualifications:

Assessor's Signature:

LOG SHEET: THEATRE PRACTICE
RULES FOR MAINTAINING ASEPSIS & STERILITY

Student Veterinary Nurse's Name:	**VN Enrolment No.:**

The evidence in this Log Sheet is a true representation of my own work.
Student Veterinary Nurse's Signature:

1. Procedures to be carried out in order to maintain asepsis and sterility in theatre:

a. Daily

● Damp dust all surfaces.

● Ensure equipment is sterile and ready to use.

● Tables are cleaned in between operations with disinfectant.

b. Weekly

● All walls and floors are thoroughly cleaned and disinfected.

● A T.S.T sterilising indicator tape is placed in each kit.

● Furniture is moved to clean thoroughly.

● Lights are disinfected.

c. Monthly

● All equipment is checked and cleaned.

● Swabs are taken then cultured for evidence of pathogens.

● The sterile equipment is checked to see if out of date.

2. Protocol to be adopted in theatre for maintaining asepsis:

a. Pre-operatively

- All equipment sterilised beforehand.
- Table disinfected.
- Surfaces are damp dusted.

b. During operations

- All contaminated material disposed of correctly.
- Care taken by surgeon and assistants not to break sterility.

c. Post-operatively

- All waste disposed of.
- Gross contamination cleaned.
- Table and surfaces disinfected.
- Floor cleaned.

Student's Comments:

The protocol is necessary to reduce the possibility of infection in the surgical wounds.

Assessor's Statement

The student nurse has demonstrated that s/he is able to maintain an aseptic environment during surgical procedures.

Comments:

Assessor's Name: **Date:**

Assessor's Qualifications:

Assessor's Signature:

LOG SHEET: THEATRE PRACTICE

MAINTAINING EQUIPMENT

Student Veterinary Nurse's Name:	VN Enrolment No.:

The evidence in this Log Sheet is a true representation of my own work.

Student Veterinary Nurse's Signature:

1. Give details of the equipment used:

Diathermy

2. State the make of equipment used in your practice

Ellman

3. Describe the procedure for the cleaning and maintenance of this equipment:

The unit is wiped clean using disinfectant.

The diathermy handpiece is detached and cleaned to remove tissue deposits. The handpiece may then be sterilised separately. The unit is electrically tested yearly.

4. Describe the procedure for sterilisation of the equipment (if appropriate):

The handpiece is placed in an autoclave bag and sterilised on low cycle (121°C) in the autoclave.

5. State THREE faults that may occur with this development:

- Electrical failure

- Fuse failure

- Handpiece becomes unplugged

6. Give details of the action that should be taken in the event of malfunction:

- Check electrical supply – refer to manufacturer

- Change fuse

- Check all leads attached correctly

Student's Comments:

The diathermy unit is used regularly and is situated within the theatre.

As well as sterilising the handpiece, it is also necessary to keep the unit clean.

Assessor's Statement

The equipment described is reflective of that in use in this training centre.

The student nurse is competent to:
- prepare it for use;
- clean and sterilise it (as appropriate); and
- identify and report malfunction (as appropriate).

Comments:

Assessor's Name: **Date:**

Assessor's Qualifications:

Assessor's Signature:

LOG SHEET: THEATRE PRACTICE
MAINTAINING EQUIPMENT

Student Veterinary Nurse's Name:	VN Enrolment No.:

The evidence in this Log Sheet is a true representation of my own work.
Student Veterinary Nurse's Signature:

1. Give details of the equipment used:

Electrocardiogram

2. State the make of equipment used in your practice:

Kontron

3. Describe the procedure for the cleaning and maintenance of this equipment:

The unit can be wiped clean with a damp cloth.

The ECG clips may be detached from the leads so that they can be cleaned and sterilised if necessary. The leads can be wiped with a damp cloth.

4. Describe the procedure for sterilisation of the equipment (if appropriate):

If necessary, the ECG clips may be sterilised by autoclaving.

5. State THREE faults that may occur with this equipment:

● Power failure

● Incorrect ECG trace

● ECG clips disconnect

6. Give details of the action that should be taken in the event of malfunction:

- If the power fails, then the fuse may be checked in the plug. Most machines have a battery back-up system.

- If the trace is incorrect, then the clips should be checked to see if they are attached and have good contact with the skin. The settings on the machine may also be checked in case they had been changed previously.

- Check all clips are connected correctly.

Student's Comments:

An ECG is an essential piece of monitoring and diagnostic equipment so correct use is vital.

Assessor's Statement

The equipment described is reflective of that in use at this training centre.

The student nurse is competent to:

- prepare it for use;
- clean and sterilise it (as appropriate); and
- identify and report malfunction (as appropriate).

Comments:

Assessor's Name: **Date:**

Assessor's Qualifications:

Assessor's Signature:

LOG SHEET: THEATRE PRACTICE

MAINTAINING EQUIPMENT

Student Veterinary Nurse's Name:	VN Enrolment No.:

The evidence in this Log Sheet is a true representation of my own work.
Student Veterinary Nurse's Signature:

1. Give details of the equipment used:

Suction pump

2. State the make of equipment used in your practice

Stephens Mk II

3. Describe the procedure for the cleaning and maintenance of this equipment:

● Detach metal suction head from plastic tubing – take off tip and clean thoroughly.

● Flush through plastic tubing with water till clean.

● Remove plastic collection chamber from main unit and empty, then clean with a disinfectant (Trigene 1:20).

● Wipe down main unit with a disinfectant (Trigene 1:20).

4. Describe the procedure for sterilisation of the equipment (if appropriate):

The metal head and plastic tube attachment are sterilized by autoclave.

5. State THREE faults that may occur with this development

● The plastic tube can melt together in the autoclave and stop suction.

● The metal suction handle can become clogged with debris.

● The unit motor can break.

6. Give details of the action that should be taken in the event of malfunction:

Report directly to theatre supervisor and label machine 'broken'.

Student's Comments:

This particular piece of equipment is very useful but care has to be taken to check the tube as this is easily destroyed by autoclaving.

Assessor's Statement

The equipment described is reflective of that in use in this training centre.

The student nurse is competent to:

– prepare it for use;

– clean and sterilise it (as appropriate); and

– identify and report malfunction (as appropriate).

Comments:

Assessor's Name: **Date:**

Assessor's Qualifications:

Assessor's Signature:

ASSESSMENT SHEET: THEATRE PRACTICE
INSTRUMENTS

Student Veterinary Nurse's Name:	VN Enrolment No.:

The evidence in this Log Sheet is a true representation of my own work.

Student Veterinary Nurse's Signature:

Assessor's Statement

The student nurse is able to identify commonly used instruments for ALL of the procedures specified in the range.

Comments:

Assessor's Name:	**Date:**
Assessor's Qualifications:	
Assessor's Signature:	

INSTRUMENTS

General Surgical Kit

6 Towel Clips (Backhaus)
6 Tissue Forceps (Allis)
6 Curved Artery Forceps (Halstead)
1 Pair Straight Scissors (Mayo)
1 Pair Dissecting Forceps (McIndoe)
2 Scalpel Handles, Size 3 and 4
1 Pair of Sponge Forceps (Rampley)
10 Gauze Swabs, 10 cm ×10 cm

2 Needleholders (Mayo-Hegar)
6 Straight Artery Forceps (Halstead)
1 Pair Curved Scissors (Mayo)
1 Pair Scissors (Metzenbaum)
2 Pairs Rat-tooth Forceps (Jean or Gillies)
1 Pair of Self-retaining Retractors (Gelpis)
1 Gallipot
5 Green Cloth Drapes

'Take Away' Kit

This is a smaller kit used for minor surgical procedures. It contains all of the above except the following:

1 Pair of Gelpis
1 Gallipot

1 Pair of Sponge Forceps
5 Cloth Drapes

Small Animal Cardiac Set

6 Towel Clips (Backhaus)
2 Scalpel Handles, Size 3 and 4
1 Pair Dissecting Forceps (McIndoe or Lane)
1 Pair Straight Scissors (Mayo)
1 Pair Curved, Long Metzenbaum Scissors
6 Pairs Tissue Forceps (Allis)
6 Pairs Curved Artery Forceps (Mosquito)
8 Satinsky Vessel Clamps
1 Diathermy Handpiece
1 Large Langenbeck
1 Pair of Sponge Forceps (Rampley)

3 Needleholders (Mayo-Hegar)
2 Pairs Rat-tooth Forceps (Jean or Gillies)
1 Pair Curved Scissors (Mayo)
1 Pair Straight, Long Metzenbaum Scissors
1 Pair Scissors (Potts)
3 Pairs Tissue Forceps (Babcock)
6 Pairs Straight Artery Forceps (Mosquito)
1 Pair Lakey Forceps
1 Pair Self-Retaining Retractors (Gelpi)
1 Gallipot

Ophthalmology Instruments

Tray One (Ophthalmic):
1 Paragon No. 7 Scalpel Handle
2 Snellens Vectis
3 Pairs of Scissors   – (Mayo sharp/sharp, straight)
                        – (Pooley's fine, conjunctival, dissection)
                        – (Castroviejo's corneal scissors)
7 Pairs of Forceps   – (Castroviejo's corneal suturing)
                        – (Arruga's intra-capsule)
                        – (St Martin's corneal suturing)
                        – (Baraquer's corneal)
                        – (Graef fixation, with lock)
                        – (Foerster iris)
                        – (Paufique, micro-teeth)
2 Pairs of Fine Fixation Forceps
6 Pairs of Halstead Mosquito Artery Forceps (2 straight, 4 curved)
2 Pairs of Tissue Forceps (Allis)
3 Pairs of Needle Holders
2 Pairs of Towel Clips (Backhaus)
1 Gallipot
1 Harrison Butler Lacrimal Cannula
1 Lister Eyelid Retractor
2 Jaffe Eyelid Retractors
1 Eyelid Speculum

CASE LOG SHEET: ANAESTHESIA

Student Veterinary Nurse's Name:	VN Enrolment No.:

The evidence in this Log Sheet is a true representation of my involvement in the case described, and the work undertaken in compiling the log is my own.

Student Veterinary Nurse's Signature:

1. Case Number-Identification:

A1

2. Case Details:

Species: CANINE   Breed: CROSSBRED

Sex: FEMALE (ENTIRE)   Age: 9 YEARS   Weight: 23 KG

3. Description of animal, including general physique:

The dog was in good general health and good physical condition. TPR was within normal limits and no other abnormalities detected on auscultation of heart and lungs.

4. Operation proposed and operation performed:

Radiography of the skull (the dog had a bony swelling within the right maxilla bone).

5. Pre-operative preparation:

The dog was starved for 12 hours prior to surgery. Water was withheld from 8 a.m. on the morning of the anaesthetic. An 18 g (over-the-needle) intravenous catheter was placed in the right cephalic vein and secured with tape.

6. Risk category:

Due to the patient's age, the physical status is classed as Class II, slight risk.

7. Premedication:

Drug: Medetomidine   Dose: 0.45 mg   Route: I/V   Time: 10.15 a.m.
          hydrochloride
Drug: Dose: Route: Time:
Drug: Dose: Route: Time:
Effect of premedication: Good

8. Induction:

Drug: Propofol   Dose: 25 mg   Route:I/V   Time: 10.25 a.m.

9. Maintenance of Anaesthesia:

Intubated: **YES** / ~~NO~~   Tube Size: 9 mm   Cuffed

Anaesthetic Machine used: Arnolds

Breathing Circuit used: Magill non-rebreathing circuit

Gas flow rates: Oxygen 7.5 litres/min

10. Details of cleaning and maintenance of equipment after use:
To include: anaesthetic machine, circuits, endotracheal tube

The ET tube was cleaned thoroughly with a bottle brush and then sterilised in Virkon before being rinsed and hung up to dry

11. Date(s):
To include: full time-scale range if appropriate

29/11/99 Dog admitted for anaesthesia and radiography. Sent home later that day.

Student's Comments:

We used a combination of Domitor and Rapinovet so that the animal recovered quickly and was able to go home.

Assessor's Statement

The procedures and details associated with the anaesthetic record described, have been observed by me and have been carried out correctly and competently:

Comments:

Assessor's Name: **Date:**

Assessor's Qualifications:

Assessor's Signature:

CASE LOG SHEET: ANAESTHESIA

Student Veterinary Nurse's Name:	VN Enrolment No.:

The evidence in this Log Sheet is a true representation of my involvement in the case described, and the work undertaken in compiling the log is my own.

Student Veterinary Nurse's Signature:

1. Case Number-Identification:

2. Case Details:

Species: CANINE   Breed: GREAT DANE
Sex: FEMALE (ENTIRE)   Age: 12 MONTHS   Weight: 54 KG

3. Description of animal, including general physique:

Dog was nervous and had snapped at a nurse and another dog. Pre-anaesthetic examination, pulse 118/minute, respiratory rate 20/minute.

4. Operation proposed and operation performed:

Investigate osteochondritis dissecans of the right shoulder joint.
Remove small particles of bone/cartilage from joint.

5. Pre-operative preparation:

Food was removed at 8 p.m. rounds the night before surgery. Water was left in kennel until premedication. An 18 g over-the-needle intravenous catheter was placed aseptically into the left cephalic vein at the time of induction.

6. Risk category:

We do not use this type of category. In theory a young fit dog is low risk, but all anaesthesia cases are treated with the same care and attention.

7. Premedication:

Drug: Acepromazine   Dose: 2.7 mg   Route: I.M.   Time: 9.15 a.m.
Drug: Butorphenol   Dose:10.8 mg   Route: I.M.   Time: 9.15 a.m.
Drug: Dose: Route: Time:
Effect of premedication: Given 35 minutes prior to induction with good sedative effect

8. Induction:

Drug: Thiopentone sodium 2.5%   Dose: 500 mg   Route: I/V   Time: 9.40 a.m.
A good quiet induction

9. Maintenance of Anaesthesia:

Intubated: **YES** / ~~NO~~   Tube Size: 12 mm cuffed

Anaesthetic Machine used: Arnolds

Breathing Circuit used: Circle system

Gas flow rates: 1.5% Halothane, 1 litre/min Nitrous oxide, 1 litre/min Oxygen

10. Details of cleaning and maintenance of equipment after use:
To include: anaesthetic machine, circuits, endotracheal tube

The endotracheal tube was soaked in a proprietary cleaner (Rapidex) for the recommended time, cleaned with a bottle brush, rinsed and hung to dry.

11. Date(s):
To include: full time-scale range if appropriate

23/3/99 (Anaesthetised from 9.40 a.m. to 11.50 a.m.)

Student's Comments:

The dog was nervous prior to premedication. It regurgitated just prior to surgery, which may have been due to the butorphenol (which has vomiting and nausea as side effects), but with no ill effect. It recovered well and we were able to use nitrous oxide with the circle as we have a capnograph which measures carbon dioxide levels.

Assessor's Statement

The procedures and details associated with the anaesthetic record described, have been observed by me and have been carried out correctly and competently:

Comments:

Assessor's Name: **Date:**

Assessor's Qualifications:

Assessor's Signature:

CASE LOG SHEET: OTHER SPECIES – EXOTICS

Student Veterinary Nurse's Name:	VN Enrolment No.:

The evidence in this Log Sheet is a true representation of my involvement in the case described, and the work undertaken in compiling the log is my own.

Student Veterinary Nurse's Signature:

1. Case Number-Identification:

EX1

2. Case Details:

Species: ERINACEIOUS EUROPAEUS   Breed: HEDGEHOG
Sex: MALE   Age: ADULT   Weight: 1.2 KG

3. Student role & reason for presentation:

Presented after attack by other animal. Caring for hedgehog during stay and giving treatment.

4. Details of hospitalisation (to include dates):

13/7/99–17/7/99

5. Principal clinical findings:
To include: injuries, illnesses etc.

The hedgehog had several cuts to its legs and a puncture wound behind its right ear. It also had a heavy worm and tick and flea burden.

6. Case Specific:
To include: diet, housing etc.

The hedgehog was kept in a cardboard pet carrier to maintain it in a warm, dark environment. Bedding of an old towel was given which was changed frequently (as hedgehogs are very messy). Water was left in at all times. The hedgehog was given hedgehog pellets and cat food with mealworms in a shallow dish (for access) ad lib. It was a good eater and did not require help.

7. Nursing Details:
To include: any methods used to reduce stress on the animal

Hedgehogs are nocturnal and an effort was made to maintain its natural environment by housing in a dark area (pet carrier). Handling was kept to a minimum except to give antibiotic injections and flea/tick treatment (e.g. Frontline, Spot-on).

Wormer was placed in food. Injections were given when the hedgehog was rolled subcutaneously taking care by wearing protective gloves.

8. Other Information:

To include: long-term management information for clients, accommodation provided, plus details of any information sheets provided etc.

As a wild animal, no long-term care can be ensured. The hedgehog was hospitalised and treated until a place was found at a wildlife hospital for rehabilitation and release.

Student's Comments:

I nursed the hedgehog during its stay and was responsible for giving treatment and maintaining its nutritional status and body weight. Weighing daily. Hedgehogs are not pets and therefore the nursing must be as non-involved as possible to aid healing by reducing stress. This had to be counterbalanced with the need to check on the hedgehog's progress.

Assessor's Statement

The procedures and details associated with the exotic case log described, have been observed by me and have been carried out correctly and competently:

Comments:

Assessor's Name: **Date:**

Assessor's Qualifications:

Assessor's Signature:

Appendix C:
Useful names and addresses

British Veterinary Nurse Association (BVNA)
Level 15
Terminus House
Terminus Street
Harlow
Essex
CM20 1XA

College of Animal Welfare
Kings Bush Farm
London Road
Godmanchester
Huntingdon
Cambridgeshire
PE18 8LJ

Qualifications Curriculum Authority (QCA)
322 Euston Road
London
NW1 2BZ

Royal College of Veterinary Surgeons
Belgravia House
62–64 Horseferry Road
London
SW1P 2AF

Scottish Qualifications Authority (SQA)
Hanover House
24 Douglas Street
Glasgow
G2 7N8

Appendix D: Further reading

QCA (1996) *Implementing the National Standards for Assessment and Verification.* NCVQ/QCA Publications, Middlesex.

QCA (1998) *Designing NVQs/SVQs: National Occupational Standards and The Role of The Independent Assessment.* QCA Publications, Middlesex.

Further copies of the above documents can be obtained by using the QCA Publications catalogue or by contacting QCA Publications, PO Box 235, Hayes, Middlesex UB3 1HF (telephone 0181 867 3333, fax 0181 867 3233).

RCVS (1998) *Veterinary Nurse Portfolio Guidance Notes.* RCVS, London.

RCVS (1999) *Training Centre Handbook.* RCVS, London.